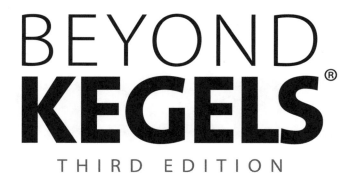

BEYOND KEGELS®

THIRD EDITION

Fabulous Four exercises and more...
to prevent and treat incontinence.

Janet A. Hulme, M.A., P.T.

Beyond Kegels, Fabulous Four exercises and more... to prevent and treat incontinence.

ISBN Number: 1-928812-17-1

Design & Layout by Michael Cutter
www.micrainbow.com

Artwork by Ed Jenne
3D Illustration by Chuck Cole

Published in the USA by
Phoenix Publishing Co.
P.O. Box 8231
Missoula, Montana 59807
www.phoenixcore.com

ACKNOWLEDGEMENTS

Many thanks to Gail Nevin, P.T., Joyce Dougan P.T., Hilary Ort P.T., Gayle Cochran Pharm.D., Judy McDonald M.D., Jane Stansbury, and Linda West R.N., for assisting in the editing of the original book. To my family, Erika, Abigail, and Richard for the time and encouragement to write. To the master editor for directing the final product. To all my patients for providing essential information about what works and more importantly what does not.

In this third edition there are many more thank-you's to offer. To the physical therapists who take Beyond Kegels® classes, thank you for all the questions that lead to new insights. To Chuck Cole, thank you for the 3D animation that makes the pelvic rotator cuff function come alive. To Ed Jenne, thank you for the illustrations from the first book to the present. To Judy Mushial and Barbara Penner thank you for believing we can "Tell a Million."

Contents

Introduction

A newborn baby eliminates urine and feces at will. The bladder and bowel empty without thought or inhibition. At the end of life there is often the same pattern. But between the beginning and end of life an important control function is toileting, releasing urine and bowel movement at the appropriate time and place. Toileting is not talked about in public. Often excuses are made when someone has to use the bathroom. Occasionally the comment is made, "I laughed so hard I messed my pants," or, "I was so scared I wet my pants."

Day-to-day, being dry and in control when urine or bowel movement is released is expected in our society. It is assumed that everyone is dry as they perform their daily activities at home and in the community. If an individual experiences leaking, he/she often feels like "the only one," "the weak one," or "the inferior person." The truth is that twenty-five to thirty percent of adults 25-55 years old have experienced bowel and bladder problems at some time. One to two percent of adults leak at night. Thirty-five to forty percent of individuals over 65 who live in the community have bladder and bowel problems, and in nursing homes over seventy percent are incontinent. Even children have leaking problems. Ten to fifteen percent of children 8-16 years old have nighttime wetting problems and three to five percent have bowel dysfunction.

The idea that between birth and death we always have control of bladder and bowel function is not true. The truth is, most of us at some time in our adult life, will experience some form of uncontrolled loss of bladder and bowel control (incontinence) that interferes with our daily activities.

Twenty-nine-year-old Mary leaks when she exercises, so she wears a pad and thinks there is nothing more she can do because she had a baby two years ago and that's part of being a mother. Ruth is 59 years old and leaks when she tries to get in the door of her house after shopping. The urge to go is so great she cannot wait. "It's just part of menopause," she tells herself. Eighty- six-year-old Barron describes explosions of urine and some leaking when he is gardening or mowing his lawn. "It's part of getting so old and still being active," he tells his daughter as he refuses to see a doctor. The idea that there is nothing to be done for leaking or incontinence is not true. A relatively simple evaluation by a health practitioner can indicate the appropriate level of treatment to eliminate the leaking in most cases. Medication, exercise, and biofeedback are the first treatments of choice. Surgery is needed for some more complicated conditions.

It is important that the individual experiencing bladder and bowel dysfunction begins by telling someone else about the problem. It may be a family member or friend at first. Just not keeping it a secret anymore is a big step. The next step is telling a health practitioner the details of the problem so an appropriate solution can be found.

In most cases exercise and self care routines are essential components of the solution to incontinence. In many cases exercise and self care routines, if adhered to on a regular basis, will eliminate the dysfunction.

The primary purpose of this book is to describe and give rationale for the Beyond Kegels® Protocol to prevent or eliminate incontinence. The Beyond Kegels® Protocol includes therapeutic exercise, autonomic nervous system training and lifestyle changes. Additional information on health professionals, evaluation procedures and medications, is discussed.

The Beyond Kegels® Protocol can be used as part of a general fitness exercise routine to prevent chronic incontinence problems. It is designed to significantly decrease or eliminate incontinence in those individuals who experience leaking caused by pelvic muscle dysfunction or bladder or bowel irritability. Exercises for incontinence are part of a total program of life-style change, physical fitness, education, and medication or surgery as indicated by special testing.

It is important to exercise under the guidance of a health care professional and to have an evaluation of the problem by a physician before starting any program.

The Program's History

The Beyond Kegels® name came about after a significant number of individuals being treated for incontinence stated that Kegel exercises did not help them to return to bladder and bowel health and control. The Beyond Kegels® program was developed to improve results from using Kegel exercises for urinary leaking. Kegel exercises were initially described by Arnold Kegel MD as contractions of the vaginal or pelvic floor muscles to stop urine flow. Kegel exercises were very helpful for some people, however many people found them difficult to understand and did not know if they were performing them correctly. Looking more completely into the structure and function of the pelvic muscles it was discovered that the support system for the bladder was more than the pelvic floor muscle. The support system was actually a combination of muscles extending through the lower pelvis and out to the leg (femur) bones. From this information the new Beyond Kegels® exercise program, designed to stimulate action of the correct pelvic muscle combination, was developed. Our experience has covered 30 years specializing in the treatment of patients with bladder and bowel health problems.

The Program's Start

Treatment began with two female nurses. One worked in an urologist's office and the other in an obstetrician's office. Both were in their early 30's. One started leaking after the birth of twins 18 months previously. The other began leaking in her 20's after she became a regular jogger and aerobics instructor. The leaking worsened after she experienced a serious illness and constant coughing. One commented, "I've tried Kegels and they haven't worked." The other nurse said, "I don't have much time for exercises. I am too busy with work and my family." At the clinic the new concepts were explained and they

4

were asked to try the new exercises. They were shown the Beyond Kegels® Protocol and agreed to try it for a few weeks. Much to their amazement both women improved significantly during the two-week period. They commented that there was decreased leaking and more confidence during daily activities.

The next person to try the Beyond Kegels® program was a 72 year old man who had a radical prostatectomy two years previously and was leaking all the time. He used the program for six weeks and experienced significant improvement. The clinic then began using the Beyond Kegels® Protocol for all patients. In six years results were compared with results from the general Kegels exercise program.

Research

Research results by Hulme and Nevin ('99) demonstrated the Beyond Kegels® Protocol to be more effective than traditional Kegel exercises. (Fig. 1-1) More individuals were completely dry using the Beyond Kegels® program and the positive results were accomplished in approximately half the time of the traditional Kegel exercises.

Sixty one percent of the people using the Beyond Kegels® program were dry in 3.5 weeks. Forty-eight percent of the people doing Kegels were dry in an average of 6.5 weeks.

In nursing home patients, the number of incontinence episodes and pads used decreased with use of the Beyond Kegels® Protocol (Penner, B and Hulme, J '99).

Penner ('02) found 100% improvement and 70% continence in a study of 43 women with stress, urge or mixed incontinence after a 4 week home program of Beyond Kegels®. Thane, M and Fegely, T ('02) reported significant improvement in individuals with recent strokes.

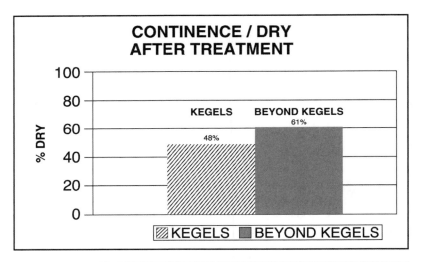

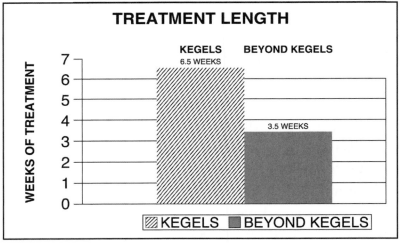

Figure 1

The program has been effective with men, women and children. It is effective with:

- children experiencing bed-wetting
- women during pregnancy and after delivery
- women during the menopausal years
- men after radical prostatectomy surgery
- men with benign prostate hyperplasia (non-cancerous prostate enlargement).

The elderly, age 70 to 95, have been helped in maintaining their independence with bladder and bowel health by using the Beyond Kegels® Protocol. It has been shown to be effective in individuals with medical problems such as multiple sclerosis and Parkinson's; after stroke and total hip replacement; and in the first levels of dementia.

Hulme J., Nevin G. *Comparison of Traditional Kegel Exercises with Obturator Internus Protocol for Treating Bladder Incontinence.* Presented at: the American Physical Therapy Association Combined Sections Meeting February 3-7, 1999; Seattle, WA.

Penner B., Hulme J. *The Effects of a Bowel and Bladder Continence Program in Incontinent Skilled Nursing Home Clients.* Presented at: the American Physical Therapy Association Combined Sections Meeting, February 3-7, 1999; Seattle, WA.

Penner B. *Outcomes of a Home Program Intervention for Urinary Incontinence - A Case Series.* Presented at: the American

Physical Therapy Association Combined Sections Meeting, February 20-23, 2002; Boston, MA.

Thane M., Fegely T. *Outcomes of Intervention for Urinary Incontinence in Hospitalized Individuals Experiencing Cerebral Vascular Accidents*. Presented at: the American Physical Therapy Association Combined Sections Meeting, February 20-23, 2002, Boston, MA.

CHAPTER 2

How Do I Determine if There is a Problem?

Any bladder or bowel activity that results in lifestyle alterations, emotional changes or feelings of discomfort is a problem. Identifying the specific characteristics and their severity is the first step in finding a solution.

History Questions

An accurate history will help to define a specific type of incontinence that then allows for appropriate treatment. Write down answers to the following questions:

General Questions

1. What is the problem in your own words?

2. How long have you had this problem?

3. How often do you experience the problem- per day, per week, per month?

   The more frequent the problem (leaking, urgency/frequency, constipation), the greater the impact on your lifestyle.

4. How much fluid do you consume daily?
   What types of fluid?
   # 8 oz. glasses_____
   Types of fluids_____
      Adequate fluid is needed and limiting fluids is
   often the first way you try to control the problem.
      Caffeinated fluids can be irritating to the bladder, bowel and nervous system.

5. What type of pads/protection do you use?
   How many per day? How many per night?
   Types_____
   # per day_____ # per night_____
      Pads/protection is one indicator of the severity of the
   problem and can be an indication of improvement.

6. What medications do you use? _____
      Some medications can cause or increase bladder
   and bowel dysfunction.

7. Do you experience any back pain, pelvic pain, leg
   or foot pain? Type of pain_____
      Back, pelvic, leg and foot pain frequently accompany bladder and bowel dysfunction especially
   when pelvic muscles and nerves are involved.

8. Do you experience any balance problems such as
   falling, tripping, using a cane or walker, using a
   handrail for stair climbing? _____

Balance problems frequently accompany bladder and bowel dysfunction when pelvic muscles and nerves are involved.

Bladder Health Questions
How can I tell what my problem might be?
When you have concerns about your bladder health or toileting habits answering the following questions can help you understand what the problem may be.

Instructions. Check all that apply.

Stress Incontinence:
1. How do you describe your problem?
☐ Leaking with physical activity, coughing or sneezing.

2. How have you changed your life because of the bladder problem?
☐ Limits physical, recreational, social activities.

Urge Incontinence:
1. How do you describe your problem?
☐ Leaking with sudden uncontrolled urge feeling.

2. Do you have trouble getting to the bathroom in time?
☐ Unable to get to the bathroom in time.

3. Have you changed your life because of the bladder problem?

☐ Frequent toileting to prevent leaking; know where every bathroom is when out of the house; limit trips and entertainment.

Functional Incontinence:

1. How do you describe your problem?

☐ Leaking occurs when unable to use toilet in a timely fashion due to mobility problems, dexterity problems, environmental factors.

2. Have you changed your life because of the bladder problem?

☐ Use a bed pan, urinal, pads, adaptive clothing, adaptive equipment or assistance.

Overflow Incontinence:

1. How do you describe your problem?

☐ Leaking occurs from a lazy bladder that does not contract well to push all urine out and/or a blocked bladder outlet that does not allow urine to flow out completely. Urine leaks out slowly and inappropriately.

2. Have you changed your life because of the bladder problem?

☐ Limit physical, recreational, and social activities.

Neurogenic Incontinence:

1. How do you describe your problem?

☐ Leaking and urine retention as a result of uncoordinated action between the bladder and bladder closure mechanisms.

2. Do you have a diagnosis of a neurological problem, ie. stroke, multiple sclerosis, Parkinson's disease, spinal cord injury?

☐ Central neurological problems affect bladder function.

Urgency and Frequency (Overactive Bladder):

1. How do you describe your problem?

☐ Little or no leaking but toileting every 1-2 hours compared to the normal every 3-4 hours in response to the feeling of urgency or the fear of leaking.

2. Have you changed your life because of the bladder problem?

☐ Toileting "just in case" you might leak.

Bowel Health Questions
How can I tell what my problem might be?

When you have concerns about your bowel health or toileting habits answering the following questions can help you understand what the problem may be.

Instructions. Check all that apply.

Constipation:

1. How do you describe your problem?

☐ Two or fewer bowel movements a week, hard bowel movements, straining to eliminate, feeling of incomplete evacuation.

2. Have your changed your life because of the bowel problem?

☐ Limit physical and recreational activities due to discomfort.

Diarrhea:
1. How do you describe your problem?
☐ Frequent passage of unformed soft to liquid stool.
2. Have you changed your life because of the bowel problem?
☐ Limit physical and recreational activities due to fear of leaking.

Irritable Bowel Syndrome (IBS)
1. How do you describe your problem?
☐ Alternating constipation and diarrhea, bloating, gas, abdominal discomfort
2. Have you changed your life because of the bowel problem?
☐ Limit physical and recreational activities due to discomfort. Dietary changes in attempt to improve symptoms.

Fecal Soiling
1. How do you describe your problem?
☐ Staining in underwear with liquid and small to large pieces of stool.
2. Have you changed your life because of the bowel problem?
☐ Isolation in fear of odor or losing control when in public.

For Women
1. Does your menstrual cycle affect bladder or bowel function?
2. How many pregnancies, miscarriages, episiotomies, vaginal deliveries and/or cesarean births have you had?
3. Were there any complications during pregnancy or delivery?
4. Did you experience leaking during or after pregnancy?
5. Have you been through or are you going through menopause?
6. Did menopause change your toileting patterns?
7. Have your been diagnosed with bladder, uterus or bowel descent?
8. Have you had a hysterectomy?

For Men
1. Have you been diagnosed with benign prostate hyperplasia (BPH)?
2. Have you been diagnosed with prostate cancer?
3. Have you had a radical prostatectomy?

Questions of Concern
Check with your health care professional.
1. Do you experience pain or discomfort in the abdominal or pelvic regions when toileting?
2. Is there blood in your urine or bowel movement (reddish to brown color)?
3. Do you have problems emptying your bladder or

bowel completely?
4. Do you have problems starting your urine flow?
5. Do you experience sudden and extreme increased urination?
6. Do you experience any rectal bleeding?

Now summarize the results of the history in a paragraph of six or seven sentences.

Normal Bladder Function
Adult bladder function is considered normal when:
1. Toileting every 2-4 hours during the day.
2. Presence of controllable awareness of need to toilet on a 2-4 hour basis.
3. Strong, continuous flow of urine for 10-20 seconds duration.
4. Urine is light yellow color and without strong odor.
5. Easy initiation and automatic completion without dribbling.
6. Absence of any leaking with physical activities, coughing, sneezing, bending, lifting, exercise, getting up from sitting and reclining.
7. Absence of frequent uncontrollable urge feelings.
8. Sleeping through the night 7-8 hours without toileting.

Exceptions to the above guidelines include:
1. Pregnancy when toileting will increase in frequency due to increased urine from the fetus and increased pressure on the bladder.

2. Aging when after 65 years of age frequency day and night increases.

Normal Bowel Function

Adult bowel function is considered normal when:
1. Toileting every day or every other day.
2. Bowel movement is of soft consistency.
3. Bowel movement is round and long like a small snake.
4. Toileting is completed without straining.
5. Presence of controllable awareness of need to toilet.
6. Absence of uncontrollable urge to toilet feelings.

The Bristol Stool Form Scale classifies bowel movements into seven types.

Type 1   Separate hard lumps or rocks that are hard to pass

Type 2   Sausage shaped and lumpy firm to hard

Type 3   Sausage shaped with cracks

Type 4   Sausage or snake shaped with smooth, soft surface- normal

Type 5   Soft blobs with clear-cut edges

Type 6   Fluffy pieces with ragged edges, mushy stool

Type 7   Water, no solid pieces, diarrhea

Heathon, K.W., et al (1992) Defecation frequency and timing, and stool form in the general population: a prospective study. Gut 33, 818-824.

Types of Bladder Dysfunction

Stress incontinence is defined as leaking caused by increased intra-abdominal pressure, such as while coughing, sneezing, lifting heavy objects, running or jumping. The leak is usually loss of a small amount of urine. Multiple leaks increase the total loss of urine.

Urge incontinence is defined as leaking in connection with a sudden uncontrollable need to toilet. A relatively large amount of urine is lost. Individuals describe coming home and experiencing the sudden urge and leaking as the key is put in the door or when they get to the bathroom and see the toilet. Urge incontinence may occur with running water, stepping into a shower or going out into cold weather.

Mixed incontinence is a combination of urge and stress incontinence with a combination of symptoms.

Functional incontinence is the inability to void in an appropriate place due to physical disability or mental confusion.

Overflow incontinence is leaking when the bladder does not empty completely during toileting. Leaking occurs from a lazy bladder that does not contract well to push all urine out and/or a blocked bladder outlet that does not allow urine to flow out completely. Urine leaks out slowly and inappropriately.

Neurogenic incontinence is leaking due to nervous system compromise that affects bladder function. Multiple sclerosis, Parkinson's disease, stroke and spinal cord injury cause bladder dysfunction.

Overactive Bladder (Urgency and Frequency) is little or no leaking but toileting every 1-2 hours compared to the normal every 3-4 hours in response to the feeling of urgency or the fear of leaking. Fear of leaking leads to "just in case" toileting and decreases the size of the bladder in response to smaller amounts of urine.

Types of Bowel Dysfunction

Constipation is two or fewer bowel movements a week, hard bowel movements, straining to eliminate and feeling of incomplete evacuation.

Diarrhea is frequent passage of unformed soft to liquid stool.

Irritable Bowel Syndrome (IBS) is alternating constipation and diarrhea, bloating, gas and abdominal discomfort.

Fecal Staining is staining in underwear with liquid and small to large pieces of stool.

Daily Diary

The next step is to keep a diary for several days. The diary will provide current information about bowel and bladder behavior, toileting frequency, leaking episodes, fluid intake and pad use. (Fig. 2-1)

The following diary can be copied and used. Under each day there are two-hour blocks of time. Record a "T" each time you urinate in the toilet, an "L" each time there is a small to medium leak, an "A" each time there is a large leak, an "F" each time there is an eight-ounce glass of fluid consumed and indicate if it is caffeinated by an asterisk (*), a "B" each time you have a bowel movement, a "BD" if there is diarrhea, a "BC" if there is constipation and a "P" if a new pad is used. Under comments, list activities and/or feelings that preceded leaks or abnormal bowel movements.

Summarize the diary results in a paragraph of five to seven sentences. How frequent are the toileting episodes during the day and night? How frequent are the leaking episodes? Do they occur during one part of the day more than another? Do they occur during one type of activity more than another? What is the pattern and description of bowel movements? How many glasses of fluid are consumed in a day? When is most of the fluid consumed? How much of it is caffeinated? How many pads are used during the day and night? How wet is the pad? Why is the pad changed?

Once the history and diary summary paragraphs are completed, a much clearer picture of the incontinence story is revealed. Based on this information, decisions about medical tests and appropriate treatment can be made.

Bladder/Bowel Diary

Name _____

Day_____ Date_____	Day_____ Date_____
6-8am _____	6-8am _____
8-10 _____	8-10 _____
10-12 _____	10-12 _____
12-2pm _____	12-2pm _____
2-4 _____	2-4 _____
4-6 _____	4-6 _____
6-8 _____	6-8 _____
8-10 _____	8-10 _____
10-12 _____	10-12 _____
overnight _____	overnight _____
*pads used _____	*pads used _____
comments _____	comments _____

T=toilet   *F-8oz. fluid*   **Figure 2-1**
L=small leak   **=caffeinated*
A=large leak   *P=pad*
B=bowel movement
BC=bowel movement constipation
BD= bowel movement diarrhea

21

CHAPTER 3

Does Anyone Else Have the Same Problem?

Case Studies

Nine individuals agreed to share their stories about incontinence. They tell about the characteristics of their incontinence, when it started, and what impact it had on their lives.

Each individual case has a unique history and pattern of incontinence, but there are also commonalities between the case studies. The case studies are presented with the intent that the reader may find similarities to his/her own story and be encouraged to read further for solutions to the leaking problem. After reading each case study, ask, "What similarities are there in this history and my problems?" "What differences are there?" After reading each succeeding chapter of this book, return to the case studies and ask, "How could this information apply to the problem described here?"

Each of the individuals in the case studies, under guidance of a health care professional, used the Beyond Kegels Protocol to significantly decrease or eliminate the leaking problem. In chapter 15, the interventions used and the results obtained at the completion of treatment are described. After completing the book, you can compare your recommendations with the treatment protocols that were actually used and see the results of that treatment.

Lizzie, 9 years old: Bed wetting

Lizzie is a 9 year-old girl who experiences night-time wetting (enuresis). She has been dry at night two times in her lifetime that she can remember. She attends a private school and is an accomplished student. She is also active in soccer and swimming.

Lizzie describes no problem getting to sleep or staying asleep at night. In fact, it is difficult for her to wake up enough to change the bed sheets and pajamas when she wets at night. Her mother puts clean sheets and pajamas beside her bed to use if she needs them. She describes feeling rested when she awakens in the morning.

During the day, Lizzie is dry. She toilets approximately every 2-4 hours. She has had no pain with urination and no bladder infections. There are no problems with constipation or diarrhea. She was toilet-trained for both bowel and bladder at approximately 2 years of age. Until she was about 6 years old, she had occasional problems getting to the bathroom in time during the day.

She describes worrying about wetting when she goes on swim team trips or for a sleep over with friends. She describes worrying about any odor she might have that would give her problem away at school. Her mother is concerned that Lizzie is becoming more isolated from her friends and sports teams because of the enuresis.

Mary, 29 years old: Stress Incontinence

Mary is 29 years old and began experiencing urinary leaking 15 months after the birth of her first child. The childbirth was complicated by a vaginal tear which was repaired surgically. Since that time, she leaks urine when she sneezes, coughs, or does any type of aerobic exercise in the standing position, i.e., brisk walking, running, dancing. She uses 3 pads a day. She toilets approximately every 2 hours during the day, and is up once or twice a night to toilet. Immediately after the childbirth and vaginal surgery, she had several bladder infections, but in the last 9 months she has been symptom-free.

At the present time, Mary works 6 hours a day as an accountant in addition to taking care of her daughter. She worked full-time before the childbirth and vaginal surgery. She tries to exercise at least 3 times a week for 30-45 minutes. She used to run 3-5 miles a day, but presently walks or exercises on a stationary bike.

She describes periodic back pain extending into her buttocks but not down her legs. Exercise seems to help the pain if she does it at the present level of 30-45 minutes, 3-4 days a week.

She describes being worried because the leaking is not decreasing with time. It limits her exercise, both the type of exercise she does and the length of time she can do it. She also is concerned that she will have to wear pads the rest of her life, and her image as a wife and lover is severely altered since the leaking started. Her husband has been understanding, but she feels as if she has to hide things about herself she did not before.

Erin, 32 years old: Stress Incontinence

Erin is 32 years old with a 3-year-old son and a job as an aerobics instructor at a health club. Erin teaches aerobics 3-4 times a week for 50 minutes. She works out daily, weight-lifting, running 3 miles a day, biking, or swimming. She golfs with her husband once a week and is in a golf league in the summer months.

Erin describes the leaking as having started about two years ago. It occurs as small leaks during aerobics and running. She wears a light pad during exercise. She leaks approximately three days a week.

Erin toilets every 3-4 hours. She drinks 2-3 colas a day and 2 cups of coffee in the morning. She drinks 5-6 glasses of water a day, usually while exercising. She consumes no alcohol and takes no medications.

Erin has had one pregnancy and delivery with no complications. She has regular menstrual cycles. Her body fat is 13 percent.

Erin is worried the problem leaking will increase as she gets older and if she has more children. She is planning to have at least one more child and wants to stay physically active the rest of her life.

Beth, 59 years old: Urge Incontinence

Beth is 59 years old and started leaking 3-4 years ago. It began one day when, after shopping, she could not get the house door open fast enough to get to the bathroom before leaking. She would have a sudden urge to go and could not hold it until she reached the toilet. Initially it occurred once every 2-3 weeks. Now she experiences 4-5 urge incidents a day and leaks at least 2-3 times a day. Sometimes the loss of urine is significant. She has started wearing dark pants so the wetness won't show. If she is out shopping and the bathroom is not close by the pad she wears may not always be adequate to contain the leaking.

She gets up 2-3 times a night, usually awakening with the feeling that she needs to go to the toilet. She has leaked small amounts during the night on occasion. She uses 1-2 super absorbent pads during the day, and puts a towel under her at night.

She has had no bladder infections, has not experienced any pain during toileting, and has no back pain.

She drinks 6-8 cups of caffeinated coffee a day, most of it before noon. She limits her fluid intake after noon, drinking only 1 glass of milk at dinner. She states that she needs the coffee to get going in the morning, but she limits fluid in the afternoon and evening so she won't leak.

She had a hysterectomy at age 41 without complications and experienced no leaking at that time. She had 3 vaginal deliveries with no significant complications, between 20 and 30 years of age.

She has tried medication which helped some but did not cure the problem and it made her feel "spacey" and disoriented so she quit using it. She has done Kegel exercises for the last three years but they haven't seemed to help.

Beth is worried that the leaking is increasing as she ages. She describes it limiting her social life. She goes only to the grocery stores and department stores where she knows the bathroom locations. She likes to travel but makes excuses in order to avoid vacationing with friends because she worries about her leaking and all the pads she would have to take. She likes to garden but, because the garden is far away from the house, she has frequent leaking problems when gardening. She states humorously that she feels as if the next step may be the nursing home.

Matilda, 82 years old: Mixed Incontinence

Matilda is a retired school teacher who describes leaking when she bends over, gets up from sitting, walks any distance, or places her hands under running water. She leaks at night when she gets up to go to the bathroom which is 2-3 times a night. She states the symptoms have been getting worse for the past 5 years but that she has had some leaking for at least 10 years. Matilda thought leaking was part of aging so she did not tell her doctor on her yearly visits until last year.

She lives alone in a condominium senior residence where she can cook for herself or go to a central dining room. She likes to exercise daily, walking the half-mile loop around the park on nice days, or riding the stationary bike in the exercise room of the social center. Matilda finds that the leaking is interfering with her exercise. She plays pinochle 2-3 times a week with friends at the social center or at one of their homes. She volunteers at the central dining room, taking meal tickets once a week. Her daughter's family takes her to church on Sunday and then out to dinner.

Matilda uses 2-3 super absorbent pads. She toilets every hour to try to keep from leaking. She drinks 3-4 cups of tea a day and a glass of orange juice in the morning. She does not like water.

Matilda finds that she has had to readjust her life in many ways to adapt to her leaking. She complains that she cannot go to church without getting up before the service is over to toilet. She has changed from wearing dresses to wearing sweat outfits in an attempt to get to the toilet more quickly. She likes dresses and feels sloppy in sweat suits. She complains that she cannot exercise as much because of the leaking.

Robert, 75 years old: Radical Prostatectomy

Robert was diagnosed with prostate cancer 2 years ago and had radical prostatectomy surgery 18 months ago. He had chemotherapy after surgery.

His leaking has been constant since the surgery. He does not perceive the leaking itself but feels the pad getting wet. He describes the leaking as gushes and relatively constant. He leaks less at night but uses a pad. During the day, he uses 3-4 pads.

Robert says he was shown Kegel exercises by his physician's nurse and has been exercising for the last year but has not noticed any difference in the leaking. He used to walk 2-3 miles day but no longer walks because of the leaking. Before the surgery, Robert helped at the senior center cleaning and setting up for meals. Now he leaks if he lifts tables or sweeps, so he has stopped going to the center because he feels helpless. Five years ago he married a woman 15 years his junior. They planned to travel when she retired but now that is on hold.

Robert has trouble getting a good stream flow of urine when he tries to urinate in the toilet. He has no problems with constipation or diarrhea. His general health is good and all tests are normal. His leaking is keeping him home and isolated, a contrast to the extrovert his wife says she married.

Barron, 86 years old: Urge Incontinence

Barron describes being an active, healthy individual. He rarely goes to the doctor but did consult one for the first time in 8 years because of the leaking problems he is experiencing. In the last 2 years he describes experiencing a sudden urge to urinate and an inability to get to the toilet in time, even though he is very agile and active for his age. He does not leak during daily activities unless he has not gone to the bathroom for several hours and lifts heavy objects. Of more concern is the sudden "explosion" he can experience, where the urine leaks in relatively large amounts with very little warning.

Barron keeps active caring for his own home, garden, and yard. He cooks his dinner but goes to the senior center for lunch. Barron is on the senior center board of directors and helps serve meals there as well. He walks a mile every morning after breakfast. His grandchildren live 3 hours away and he drives to see them frequently.

His physician prescribed a medication for the leaking but when Barron tried it he almost passed out. His blood pressure, which was normal before, significantly decreased.

Barron describes limiting how much he drinks and toileting every hour in an attempt to control the leaking. He experiences explosions once or twice a week. He uses a small washcloth in his underwear to absorb any leaking but says if there is a major explosion, it cannot hold it all.

Ken, 55 years old: Constipation

Ken is a 55 year-old male who has experienced constipation for many years. He has bowel movements one to two times a week. He describes straining and pushing hard to eliminate rock hard, pebble like stools. He often feels that he has not emptied completely after having a bowel movement. There is a vague discomfort in his lower abdomen but he cannot count on that feeling telling him he can have a bowel movement. He experiences urgency to urinate but no leaking. He describes hemorrhoids several times a year.

Ken describes drinking 1-2 pots of coffee a day. He drinks very little water. His favorite food is pasta with various sauces. He eats very few vegetables and no salads. He eats an apple a day and occasionally has a banana.

Ken works two jobs five days a week. He is an accounting assistant during the day and teaches bookkeeping at a community college at night. On weekends he watches college football or NASCAR on TV and occasionally goes to a sporting event. He mows the lawn and does minor home repairs but has no regular exercise program.

Ken has come to the clinic because of the difficulty with bowel movements and the increasing abdominal discomfort. Medical tests indicate chronic constipation without impaction.

Lillie, 24 years old: Diarrhea

Lillie is a 24 year-old female who experiences bouts of diarrhea on a weekly basis. She can have one to two bouts of diarrhea a day and then go for several days without a bowel movement. She has soft but formed bowel movements approximately fifty percent of the time. Lillie describes lower abdominal discomfort and increased gas. She eliminates urine three to four times a day.

Lillie describes drinking 2-3 diet caffeinated sodas and three glasses of milk a day. She eats bran cereal with pear or peach for breakfast. She eats a salad or soup for lunch. For dinner she has chicken or fish and cooked broccoli, green beans or carrots. Desserts are always of the diet variety.

Lillie works as a personal trainer in a health club. She leads aerobic exercise classes twice a day and runs 3-5 miles a day. On weekends she likes to hike or bike. The diarrhea is limiting her ability to continue these activities as she is afraid of losing control when she is exercising. She wears a pad during physical activity "just in case" she has an accident. She has experienced diarrhea once or twice while running. During aerobic classes she leaves for a few minutes if the diarrhea comes on. She is afraid this will continue to get worse.

CHAPTER 4

What Health Care Providers Can Help? What Special Tests Can Be Done?

Many people with bladder and bowel health problems do not tell anyone about the problem because they think there is nothing that can be done, or they are too embarrassed to say anything. It is important that the general public become more aware of the appropriate health care providers who can be of help to them. It is equally important that health care providers who routinely perform physical examinations and treat acute problems include bladder and bowel health questions in the history portion of the evaluation.

Primary health care providers, such as family practice physicians, general practice physicians, internists, geriatricians, physicians' assistants, and nurse practitioners, can do the initial screening for incontinence using questions in the history portion of the evaluation or on a written questionnaire. If a problem is indicated from the history, further testing can be done.

Bladder Dysfunction

As recommended in Clinical Practice Guideline, No. 2, 1996 Update published by the Department of Health and Human Services, physical examination, routinely done by a physician or other health care professional, includes the following:

1) Palpation of the abdomen for diastasis recti, masses, swelling or edema, tender or painful areas.
2) Genital examination in men to detect abnormalities of the foreskin, glans penis, and perineal skin condition.
3) Pelvic examination in women to evaluate perineal and genital skin condition, pelvic organ position, possible masses, pelvic muscle tone, etc.
4) General examination to detect possible neurological conditions such as multiple sclerosis, stroke, spinal cord compression, etc.; to assess independence of movement, mental status, and eye-hand coordination in the frail or functionally impaired; and to detect general edema or other systemic conditions.
5) Direct observation of urine loss. The individual is asked to cough strongly while the examiner observes urine loss. The test is done in supine but if no leakage is observed it is repeated in sitting and standing. If leakage occurs with coughing, stress incontinence is indicated; if leaking is delayed or persists after coughing, urge incontinence is indicated.

Additional basic tests can include:
1) Measurement of Post Void Residual Volume (PVR) using a pelvic ultrasound or catheterization. PVR is the urine left in the bladder after toileting. Before PVR is measured, the individual voids completely; the PVR is done within minutes after the voiding. It is important that the individual be

comfortable and relaxed during the voiding so the maximum urine is released before measuring the PVR. There is no documented normal PVR, but in general a PVR of 30-50 cc is considered adequate bladder emptying, and a PVR greater than 200 cc is considered retention.

2) Urinalysis is conducted to detect conditions including infection, cancer, diabetes, or kidney stones. Careful cleaning of the genitalia with an antiseptic solution allows a "clean catch" of urine that can be analyzed.

A specialist, usually a urologist, provides specialized testing when the initial work-up and treatment does not solve the problem. Urologists are trained to perform specialized tests and surgical procedures of the urogenital system. They treat the more complicated cases.

The specialized tests include urodynamic tests, endoscopic tests, and imaging tests.

Urodynamic Tests These tests are used to assess the anatomic and functional status of the bladder and urethra. When performing urodynamic testing, the urologist attempts to reproduce the individual's symptoms.

Cystometry One part of urodynamic testing is cystometry. This test measures bladder contractility with bladder filling. The bladder is filled to capacity using a urethral catheter, a plastic tube inserted in the urethra, and the action of the bladder muscle is measured as the bladder is filling.

Voiding Cystometrogram This is also called a pressure flow study. It can measure bladder contractility and pressure in the urethra as the individual urinates, which enables the evaluation of possible urethral obstruction.

Uroflowmetry This test measures the urine flow rate which may be helpful in individuals who have problems with bladder emptying. It is helpful in diagnosing some types of male incontinence.

Urethral Pressure Profilometry This measures resting pressure and dynamic pressure in the urethra. Sphincter function can also be assessed.

Electromyography This measures the nerve and muscle activity of voluntary sphincter muscles. Needle or surface electromyography can be used in association with a cystometrogram to aid in diagnosing specific types of incontinence.

Endoscopic Testing This test is performed when there is recent onset of irritable voiding symptoms, bladder pain, recurrent cystitis, a suspected foreign mass or blood in the urine without infection. The test performed is called a cystourethroscopy and is similar to an arthroscopy of the knee or shoulder joint. A miniature camera is placed in the bladder through the urethra. The urologist can assess the condition of the bladder, bladder wall, and bladder angle by observing the screen and taking video records of the test.

Imaging Tests X-ray and ultrasonographic imaging are the most common tests used for evaluation of anatomic conditions associated with urologic conditions.

Upper Tract Imaging Ultrasound of the kidneys, bladder, or both can help identify dilation of the upper urinary tract and kidney pathology.

Lower Tract Imaging This ultrasound of the urinary bladder and urethra, with and without voiding, is helpful in examining the anatomy of this area. This test can help in identifying bladder neck stability or mobility, urethral obstruction, and degree of cystocele.

Videourodynamics This technique combines the urodynamic tests with fluoroscopy and is used in complicated cases.

Bowel Dysfunction

Physical examination performed by a health care professional includes:

1) palpation of the abdomen for tenderness, tightness, pain and muscle spasm,
2) visual examination of the anal sphincter, and
3) palpation and digital examination of the anus and distal rectum for fissures, hemorrhoids, prolapse.

A specialist, usually a gastroenterologist or anorectal surgeon, provides specialized testing when the initial work-up and treatment does not solve the problem. They treat more complicated cases.

Additional tests can include:

1) flat plate abdominal x-ray to diagnose constipation and impaction,
2) proctoscopy and sigmoidoscopy to diagnose anal fissures and internal hemorrhoids,
3) flexible sigmoidoscopy and colonoscopy to diagnose polyps and tumors,

4) anorectal manometry to assess anorectal nerve and muscle function, and

5) anal ultrasound and MRI to assess tissue layers and condition.

Pelvic Muscle Dysfunction

Clinicians work with individuals experiencing incontinence in order to assess and treat any musculoskeletal component that may be a contributing factor. Dysfunction of the urogenital and pelvic diaphragm muscles often contribute to incontinence. Dysfunction of the breathing diaphragm, abdominal, hip rotator and gluteal muscles can affect bladder control. A high percentage of individuals who are experiencing incontinence also suffer from back, hip, or pelvic pain.

Accurate assessment and treatment of back or hip pain can be an important part of treating incontinence because back and hip pain can be associated with nerves innervating the pelvic region. The presence of muscle dysfunction, such as rectus diastasis or piriformis spasm, is assessed and treated by the physical therapist simultaneously with re-education of the pelvic muscles to decrease or eliminate incontinence.

Physical and occupational therapists, nurses, and psychologists with specialized training in biofeedback and incontinence evaluate and treat pelvic muscle dysfunction in connection with incontinence. Using evaluation skills ranging from observation to palpation to biofeedback, the therapist objectively quantifies the integrity of the pelvic muscles that support the internal organs of bladder, uterus, and bowel during rest and daily activities. Based on the evaluation results, the trained therapist outlines a progressive neuromuscular re-education and therapeutic exercise program designed to improve pelvic muscle function and to restore continence.

Observation

Observation of the pelvic muscles during bearing down or pushing indicates the presence and severity of a uterine prolapse, cystocele, rectocele, or enterocele. A uterine prolapse occurs when the uterus descends into the vaginal canal. A cystocele is a bulging of the bladder into a weak area of the vaginal wall. A rectocele is a bulging of the rectum into a weak vaginal wall. An enterocele is a protrusion of the pouch of Douglas into a weak vaginal wall. There are degrees of severity for each of these conditions. During pushing or bearing down, the uterus, bladder, or rectal bulge is observable through the vaginal opening in more severe cases.

Pelvic Muscle Testing

Palpation of the pelvic muscles is performed to assess strength and symmetry of the pelvic diaphragm and urogenital muscles. Two gloved fingers are inserted into the vagina or rectum to palpate muscle action. In the lithotomy position, the individual is instructed to:
1) Tighten and release the pelvic muscles quickly six times;
2) Tighten the pelvic muscles and hold for ten seconds, then release/relax them for ten seconds. Repeat six times.

Muscle strength can be graded on a 0-3 scale. (Fig 4-1)

Pelvic Muscle Strength Rating Scale:

	0	1	2	3
Pressure	None	Weak, feel pressure on side of fingers, but not all around	Moderate feel pressure all around	Strong, fingers compress/ override
Duration	None	<1 Second	1-3 Seconds	>3 Seconds
Displacment in plane	None	Slight incline, base of fingers moves up	Greater incline fingers move up along total length	Fingers move up and are drawn in

Figure 4-1

Biofeedback

Biofeedback using surface, vaginal or rectal sensors assesses the pelvic muscles' function in supine, sitting, and standing positions. Resting level, quick contractions, and ten-second hold contractions are measured in microvolts of electrical activity coming from the nerve/muscle connection. Recruitment patterns and endurance of the pelvic muscles can also be assessed. Frequently, a second channel monitors the abdominal or gluteal muscles to assess accessory muscle use during attempted pelvic muscle contractions.

Based on information obtained from the history and physical assessment an appropriate treatment protocol is developed.

CHAPTER 5

How Does My Body Work? Anatomy and Function of the Urinary, Bowel and Pelvic Muscle Systems

The structures and functions of the urogenital, gastrointestinal and pelvic muscle systems are important to understand when developing exercises to be done for bladder and bowel dysfunction. These systems must work together with the nervous system to achieve optimal bladder and bowel health.

The Pelvis

The pelvis is the scaffolding for the organs and muscles involved in continence. The right and left sides of the pelvis are each divided into three parts: 1) the ilium, 2) the ischium, and 3) the pubis. The pelvis connects posteriorly with the sacrum at the sacroiliac joints. The pelvis connects anteriorly at the symphysis pubis joint. (Fig. 5-2)

Pelvic Organs

The urogenital organs include:
1) bladder,
2) uterus and vagina in women,
3) prostate gland in men, and
4) bowel, rectum and anus. (Fig. 5-3 and 5-4)

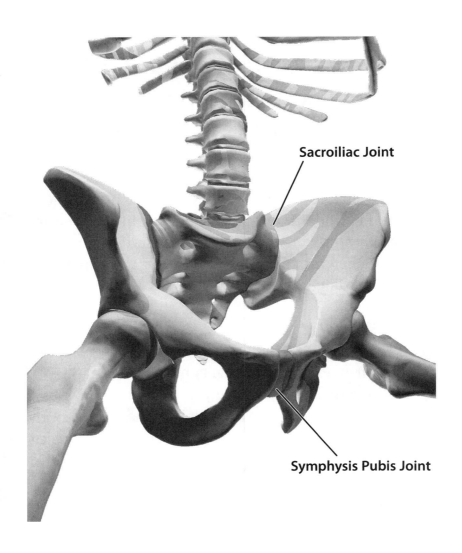

Sacroiliac Joint

Symphysis Pubis Joint

Figure 5-2

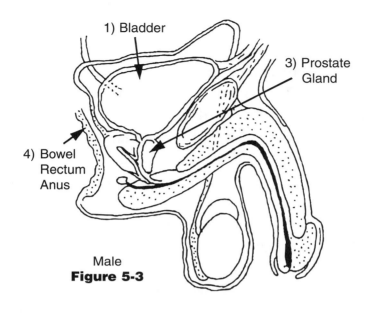

1) Bladder

3) Prostate
Gland

4) Bowel
Rectum
Anus

Male
Figure 5-3

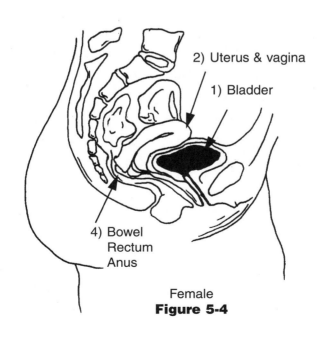

2) Uterus & vagina

1) Bladder

4) Bowel
Rectum
Anus

Female
Figure 5-4

43

The bladder is located just behind the pubic symphysis and tips forward toward the symphysis pubis. The uterus is positioned just behind the bladder. It also tips forward and helps to maintain the forward position of the bladder. The bladder angle is the angle between the bladder and the urethra. It acts like a bend in a straw to keep urine in the bladder. The prostate gland in men surrounds the urethra close to the bladder neck.

The bowel, rectum, and anus are positioned just behind the uterus. The anorectal angle is the angle between the anus and rectum. It helps to keep the bowel movement in the intestines until it is time to toilet.

Fascial and Ligamentous Support

There is fascial and ligamentous support to maintain the bladder, uterus, and bowel in optimal position for function.

The urethropelvic ligaments stabilize and are the major support for the bladder neck and proximal urethra. These fibers surround the bladder neck and proximal urethra and extend laterally to the obturator tendon bilaterally. This ligament transfers forces from the pulley system of the obturator internus and obturator tendon to facilitate bladder elevation and support of the bladder neck. (Fig.5-5)

The pubourethral ligaments support and stabilize the mid-urethra. They attach to the pubic bone and surround the mid-urethral region. (Fig.5-6)

The periurethral fascia is a continuation of the ligamentous support and stabilization connecting the urethra and vagina. (Fig.5-7)

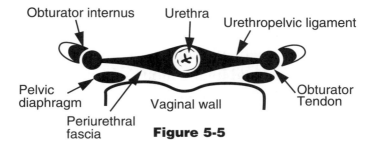

Figure 5-5

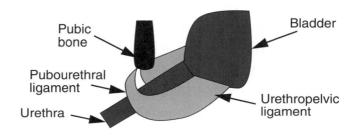

Figure 5-6

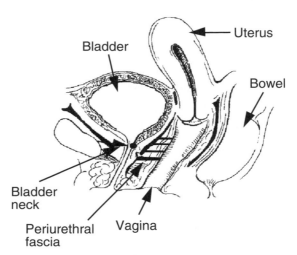

Figure 5-7

45

As the obturator internus muscles contract they increase tension on the obturator tendon which elevates the bladder via the urethropelvic ligament, periurethral fascia, and pelvic diaphragm.

These fascial and ligamentous supportive structures help to maintain the bladder positioned up in the pelvis, the bladder neck stabilized, and the angle of the bladder and uterus forward toward the pubic bone. (Fig.5-7)

The Urinary System

The structures of the urinary system include:
1) two kidneys,
2) two ureters,
3) bladder or detrusor muscle, and
4) urethra. (Fig. 5-8)

The kidneys produce urine which is transported through the ureters to the bladder, a hollow muscular organ. The bladder expands to hold approximately one pint of fluid. It contracts to force the urine through the urethra to the outside.

The urethra, a hollow, muscle-lined tube is approximately the length of a thumb (5cm) in the female and the length of a straw (20cm) in males. The smooth muscle lining of the urethra maintains relatively high resting tone to keep urine in and relaxes to let urine flow out. The urethra is richly lined with mucous glands and blood vessels which produce fluids that cause the urethral surfaces to stick together at rest. This is called coaptation. At rest, when not urinating, the urethra is a

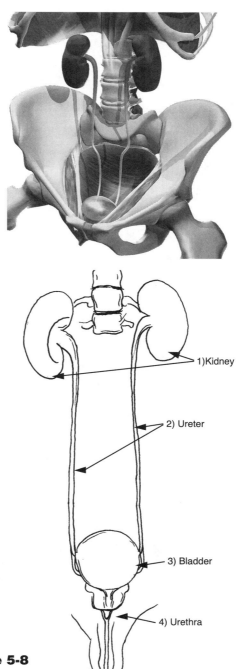

1) Kidney

2) Ureter

3) Bladder

4) Urethra

Figure 5-8

47

collapsed tube closed by coaptation and smooth muscle resting tone.

The Gastrointestinal (Bowel) System

The structures of the gastrointestinal system include:
1) mouth and esophagus
2) stomach
3) small intestine
4) large intestine and colon
5) rectum and anus. (Fig. 5-9)

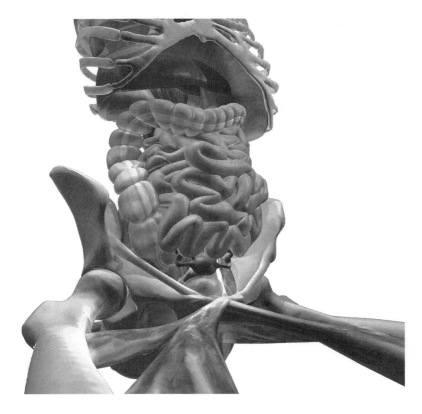

Figure 5-9

The mouth and teeth pulverize the food you eat and transfers that food down the esophagus to your stomach. In your stomach digestive juices continue to breakdown the food into chemical compounds. Then these nutrients are emptied into the small intestine. In the small intestine nutrients combine to form the building blocks that repair and replace all cells in your body and to form the chemical messengers that regulate and control all body functions. The building blocks and chemical messengers are released through nerve transmission and through the blood stream. The remaining material is transferred to the large intestine and colon where water is absorbed back into the body. As the feces is transferred to the rectum and anus messages to the brain tell you it is time to have a bowel movement.

As the colon moves the feces into the lower colon and rectum the internal sphincter relaxes. The external sphincter and pelvic diaphragm loop increases in tone to improve two main closure mechanisms of the sphincter and anorectal angle that keep your bowel movement in your body until you are on the toilet.

The Skeletal Muscles

The skeletal muscles important in Beyond Kegels® exercises include:

1) breathing diaphragm,
2) pelvic diaphragm/levator ani,
3) urogenital diaphragm/perineum,
4) external sphincter,
5) obturator internus (hip rotators),
6) abdominals (stomach), and
7) adductors.

The Breathing Diaphragm Muscle

The breathing diaphragm muscle sits below the ribs attaching to the sternum, ribs, and thoracic-lumbar spine. (Fig.5-10) During inhalation, the breathing diaphragm pulls down like a shade pulling over a window. It compresses the abdominal contents and increases pressure on the bladder and bowel (increases intra-abdominal pressure). During exhalation, the breathing diaphragm returns to the dome shape, decreasing intra-abdominal pressure. The breathing diaphragm is a voluntary muscle controlled primarily by the autonomic nervous system.

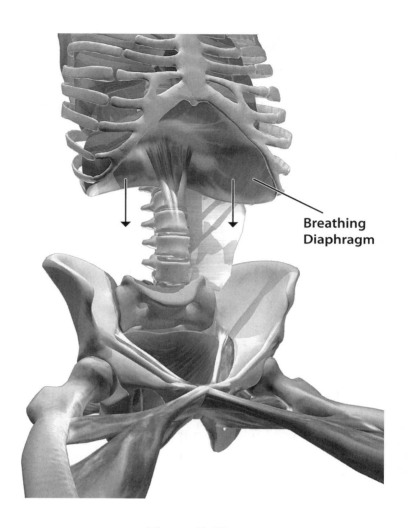

Breathing
Diaphragm

Figure 5-10

51

The Pelvic Diaphragm/Levator Ani Muscles

The pelvic diaphragm, also known as the levator ani, supports and stabilizes the internal organs of the bladder, uterus, and bowel. The pelvic diaphragm attaches to the obturator tendon (tendinous arch), the pubis and the sacrum. (Fig. 5-11) During contraction of the pelvic diaphragm/levator ani, there is increased support and stabilization of the bladder and bowel. There is improved closure of the urethral and anal sphincters. (Fig.5-12)

The three muscles forming the pelvic diaphragm include:

1) pubococcygeus,
2) iliococcygeus, and
3) ischiococcygeus or puborectalis

These muscles form a bowl of loops running front to back in the pelvis. The slings have relatively high resting tone. This constant tone at rest helps to keep the bladder and bowel outlets closed until it is time to go to the bathroom.

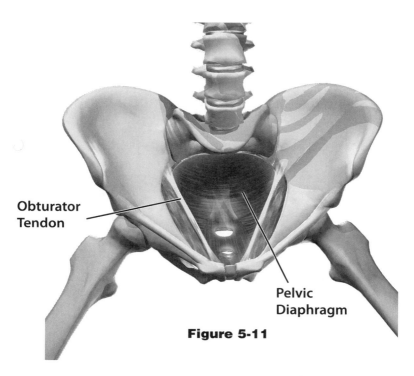

Obturator
Tendon

Pelvic
Diaphragm

Figure 5-11

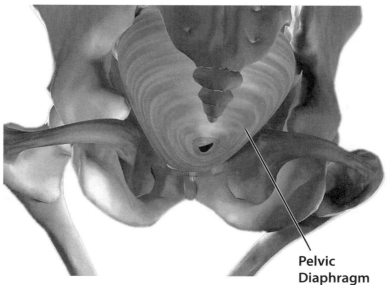

Pelvic
Diaphragm

Figure 5-12

53

The Urogenital Diaphragm Muscles

The urogenital diaphragm is the more superficial of the diaphragm muscles. (Fig.5-13) It attaches to the symphysis pubis, pubic rami, the perineal body and the ischial tuberosities.

The urogenital diaphragm is composed of a triangle of three muscles. It includes:

1) transverse perineal,
2) bulbospongeosus or bulbocavernus, and
3) ischiocavernus

This group of muscles interdigitates with the pelvic diaphragm and external anal sphincter via fascia and the perineal body.

The urogenital diaphragm primarily assists with sexual function and urethral sphincter action. It contracts quickly and forcefully. It fatigues quickly.

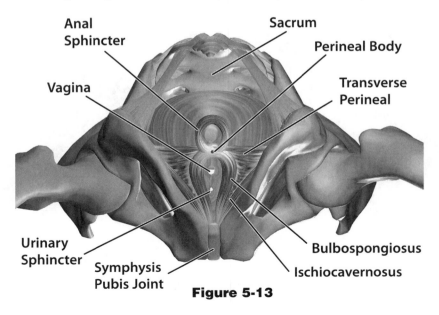

Figure 5-13

Fast and Slow Twitch Fibers

Muscle fibers of the pelvic and urogenital diaphragms are divided into two types.

Fast twitch fibers, approximately 35%, act fast and intensely when coughing, sneezing, or doing something else unexpected that increases the pressure on the urethra. These fibers are like the leg muscles used during a sprint; they are powerful, explosive, and fatigue relatively quickly. The urogenital diaphragm muscles are primarily fast twitch fibers used to stop sudden urine release.

Slow twitch fibers, approximately 65%, act at a slow, constant tone for postural support. These fibers are like the calf muscles that maintain upright posture by contracting at a constant, low level. The pelvic diaphragm muscles are primarily slow twitch fibers supporting the bladder and urethra in optimum position for continence.

The pelvic and urogential diaphragm muscles act together somewhat like a hammock. In the resting position they gently support the internal organ structures. During physical activity or when there is a need to urinate and the toilet is not readily available, their resting tone increases much like a hammock pulls up and in when someone reclines in it. This hammock helps prevent leaking. (Fig. 5-14)

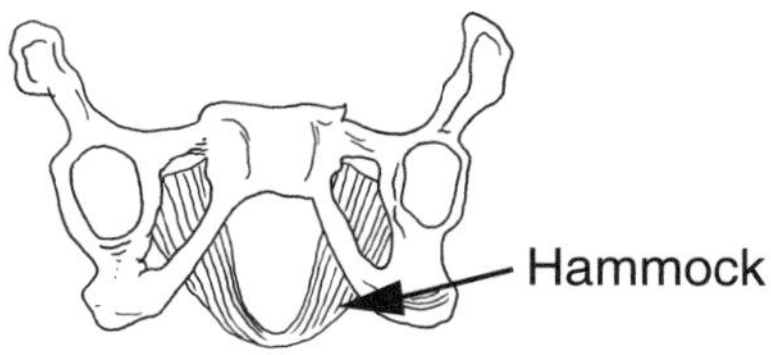

Figure 5-14

The Sphincter Muscles

The sphincter muscles include:

1) external urinary and anal sphincters, and
2) internal urinary and anal sphincters. (Fig. 5-15)

The urinary and anal sphincters are circular muscles similar to your mouth, the obicularis oris muscle. These muscles can tighten to pucker and relax to open. They are the only muscles in the body that do not attach to any bone but rather are suspended in space and attach to other muscles. The urinary sphincter attaches to the urogenital diaphragm muscles. The anal sphincter

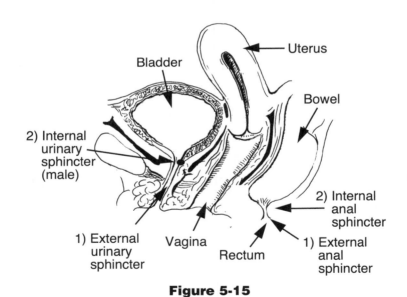

Figure 5-15

56

attaches to the pelvic diaphragm and urogenital diaphragm muscles. When the urogenital diaphragm and
pelvic diaphragm contract they change the tone and
action of the urinary and anal sphincters.

The external sphincters are controlled by the voluntary and autonomic nervous systems. An individual
can relax and tighten these circular muscles. Most of
the time the external sphincters are resting closed as
directed by the autonomic nervous system.

The internal urinary sphincter in males and the bladder angle in females, and the internal anal sphincter in
male and female, serve the same function but are not
under our voluntary control. (In the female, the bladder
angle functions as the internal urinary sphincter since
an actual sphincter is not present.)

Obturator Internus Muscle

Each of the two obturator internus muscles covers the obturator foramen within the pelvis attaching around its borders and to the obturator (arcuate) tendon on each side. (Fig.5-16) It travels out of the pelvis via the lesser sciatic notch to attach on the posterior aspect of the greater trochanter of the femur (leg bone). A pulley action occurs at the lesser sciatic notch where the obturator internus turns a 120 degree angle as it exits the pelvis. (Fig. 5-17)

The obturator internus muscle attaches on the lateral aspect and the pelvic diaphragm attaches on the medial aspect of the obturator tendon. The urethropelvic ligament and periurethral fascia which support the bladder and urethra surround the pelvic diaphragm/levator ani and also attach to the obturator tendon. So, as the oburator internus contracts, it acts as a pulley lifting the bladder and urethra into position for optimum function through the obturator tendon, pelvic diaphragm and fascial/ligamentous connections. The resting length and tone of the obturator internus muscle also effects the bladder and bowel position in the pelvis.

The obturator internus muscles function to:
1) rotate the legs out from midline,
2) facilitate increased pelvic and urogenital diaphragm muscle tone, and
3) lengthen adductors.

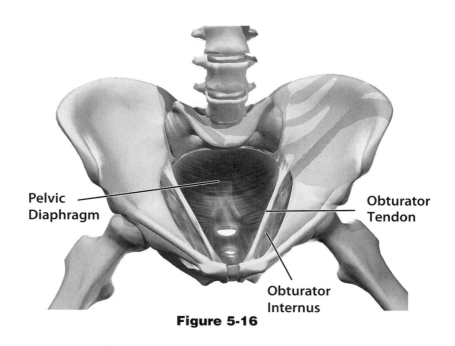

Pelvic
Diaphragm

Obturator
Tendon

Obturator
Internus

Figure 5-16

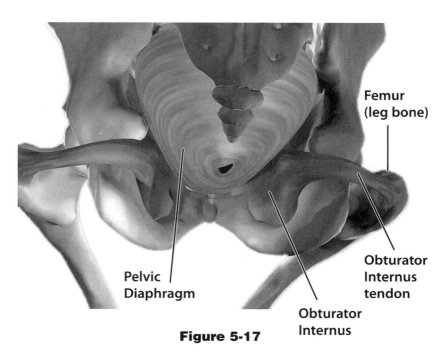

Femur
(leg bone)

Obturator
Internus
tendon

Pelvic
Diaphragm

Obturator
Internus

Figure 5-17

59

Adductor Muscles

The adductor muscles attach to the pelvis at the pubic rami close to the attachment of the urogenital and pelvic diaphragm muscles and along the shaft of the femur. (Fig. 5-18) The adductor muscles function to:

1) bring the legs toward each other,
2) facilitate pelvic and urogential diaphragm muscle tone, and
3) lengthen the obturator internus.

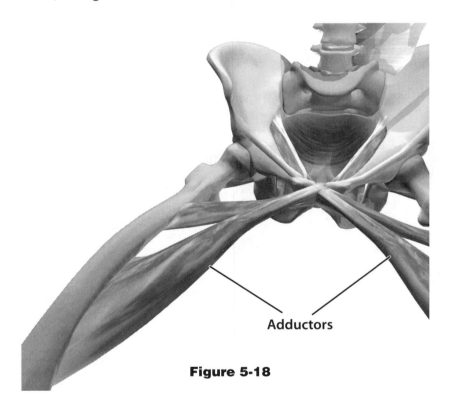

Adductors

Figure 5-18

60

Abdominal Muscles

The abdominal muscles are attached to the ribs, the sternum, and the pubic bone. (Fig. 5-19) They contract during lifting, pushing, and during rigid postural stance. During contraction, they increase intra-abdominal pressure, which increases pressure on the bladder, pelvic and urogenital diaphragm muscles.

The transverse abdominus muscle automatically contracts with the pelvic muscles facilitating their action. If the abdominal muscles are chronically contracted, the breathing diaphragm cannot descend during inhalation. If the abdominal muscles are chronically contracted, there is constant pressure on the bladder, which can lead to bladder irritability and urge incontinence.

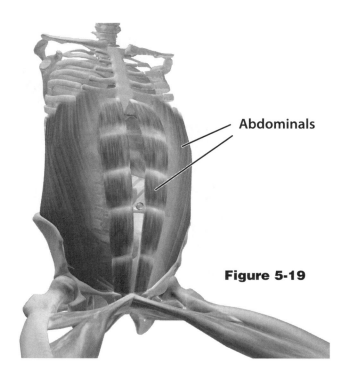

Abdominals

Figure 5-19

Gluteal Muscles

The gluteal muscles attach to the posterior aspect of the pelvis and the sacrum as well as the femur (thigh). They are frequently tightened when attempting to contract the pelvic and urogenital diaphragm muscles to control leaking. Because they are a large muscle group, they can overpower the pelvic muscles, so the gluteal muscles should be relaxed during most exercises dealing with incontinence. (Fig. 5-20)

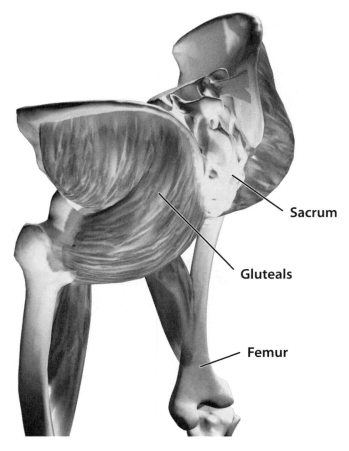

Sacrum

Gluteals

Femur

Figure 5-20

Nervous Systems Involved in Bladder and Bowel Control

There are two types of nervous systems involved in bladder control: the voluntary nervous system and the autonomic or automatic nervous system. (Fig. 5-21)

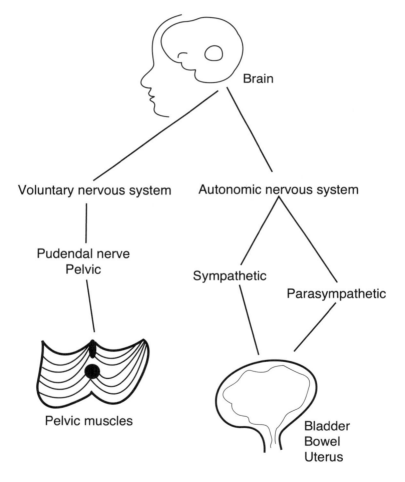

Figure 5-21

The Voluntary Nervous System

The voluntary nervous system, from sacral nerve roots 2, 3 and 4 (1) , sends and receives information from the pelvic and urogenital diaphragm and external sphincter muscles (2) via the pudendal nerve (3) . (Fig. 5-22) This enables an individual to tighten and release these muscles on command. It is possible, by tightening the muscles, to strengthen them through exercise, because the nerves tell the muscles what to do through the voluntary nervous system.

The Autonomic Nervous System

The autonomic nervous system controls the bladder and bowel during filling and emptying. The autonomic nervous system has two divisions that originate from the subcortex and travel down the spinal cord to their target organs. The sympathetic division nerve roots exit from vertebrae at the thoracic and lumbar spine. The parasympathetic division nerve roots exit from vertebrae at the cranial and sacral spine. (Fig.5-23)

Sympathetic nerves are both excitatory and quieting to the bladder and bowel.

One part of the sympathetic system controls closure of the bladder outlet. (A) A second part of the sympathetic system controls relaxation of the bladder wall while the bladder fills with urine. (B) A third part of the sympathetic system controls resting tone of the pelvic muscles so they support the bladder and bowel in the pelvis and maintain the urinary and anal sphincters closed. (C) The sympathetic nervous system primar-

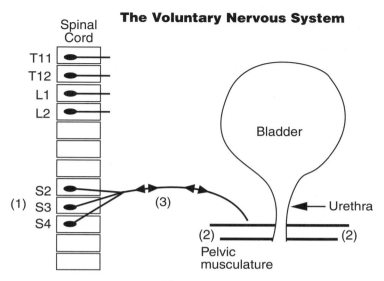

The Voluntary Nervous System

Figure 5-22

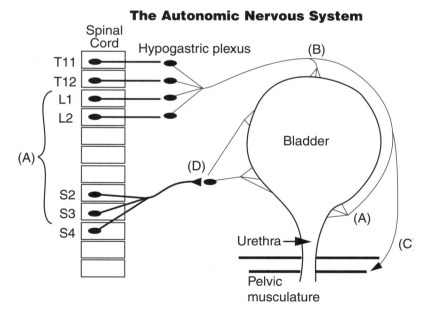

The Autonomic Nervous System

Figure 5-23

65

ily quiets the gut slowing the movement of the feces through the colon.

Parasympathetic nerves are primarily excitatory to the bladder and bowel. One part of the parasympathetic system stimulates bladder contractions during urination. (D) The parasympathetic nervous system primarily stimulates contraction of the gut increasing the speed of movement of the feces through the colon.

Bladder Emptying

Twelve to fourteen unconscious reflex arcs control bladder and bowel function. Bladder emptying/urination, is controlled by several automatic reflexes. (Fig. 5-24) As the bladder fills, it stretches, sending nerve messages to the brain telling how full the bladder is (1) . The brain via the autonomic nervous system sends back messages to the bladder to release at the bladder neck and urethra (2) so the urine can flow out, and to contract gently at the bladder wall (3) to push the urine out. In men, there is more active bladder contraction to push urine out. In women, it is more a release of a tightened bladder neck and urethra.

During bladder emptying, the pelvic diaphragm, urogenital diaphragm, and external sphincter muscles relax at the direction of the autonomic nervous systems (4) .

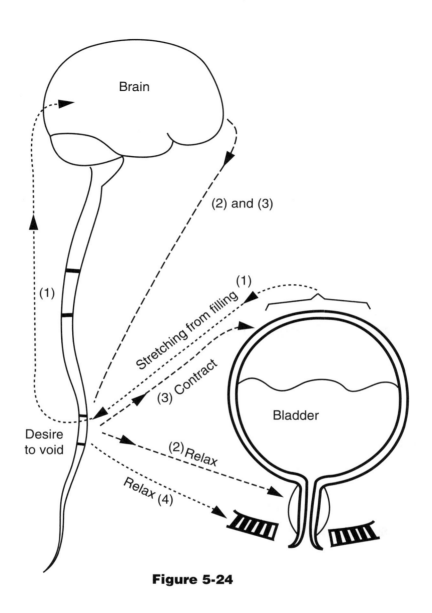

Figure 5-24

Bowel Emptying

During bowel emptying the same general pattern occurs. As the lower colon and rectum fills it stretches and messages are sent to the brain telling you that the bowel is full. The brain via the autonomic nervous system sends back messages to the colon and rectum to contract and push the bowel movement out. At the same time messages through the autonomic nervous system tell the pelvic muscle loop of the puborectalis and the external sphincter to relax to straighten the anorectal angle and open the sphincter so the bowel movement slides out without effort.

Bladder and Bowel Filling

When the bladder and bowel are empty, reflex arcs quiet the system so they can start filling again. (Fig. 5-25) The brain via the sympathetic nervous system tells the bladder to relax (1) . It stimulates the urethral closure mechanisms (2) so the urine can once more be stored in the bladder without leaking.

The pelvic muscles, stimulated by the sympathetic nervous system, return to the resting tone that maintains urethral closure (3). The resting tone of the pelvic muscles is set by the autonomic nervous system.

When the bladder and bowel are empty, reflex arcs activate the closure mechanisms of the urethra and rectum so the bladder and bowel can begin filling again. (Fig 5-25) It tells the five closure mechanisms of the urethra to automatically return to resting level closed.

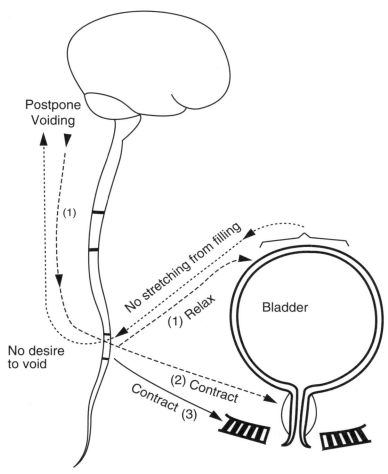

Figure 5-25

These closure mechanisms include:
1. internal and external urinary sphincters,
2. pelvic diaphragm loops,
3. bladder angle,
4. urethral smooth muscle lining, and
5. urethral coaptation- sticky goo.

The autonomic nervous system tells the three closure mechanisms of the rectum and anus to automatically return to resting level closed. These include:

1. internal and external anal sphincters,
2. pelvic diaphragm loops, and
3. anorectal angle.

Reflex Connections

There is a reflex connection between the bladder (detrusor) muscle and the pelvic muscles. (Fig. 5-26) When an individual has the urge to urinate but needs to wait, the pelvic and urogenital diaphragm muscles contract to stop the urine flow (1) . Contraction of the pelvic and urogenital diaphragm muscles sends messages to the bladder muscle telling the bladder to relax (2) , thus keeping it from losing urine before the individual gets to a bathroom. This is termed reflex inhibition.

Similar to when an individual moves his/her hand to the mouth to eat (the biceps contracts and reflexively tells the triceps to relax so the elbow can move to bring the hand to the mouth), when there is an urge to urinate the pelvic muscles contract to keep the individual dry and reflexively tell the bladder muscle to relax until the toilet can be reached.

Stress, Urge, and Mixed Incontinence

If stress incontinence is a problem, (small to moderate amounts of urine are lost when an individual jumps, runs, coughs, or sneezes), the pelvic and urogenital diaphragm muscles' tone is not adequate to overcome

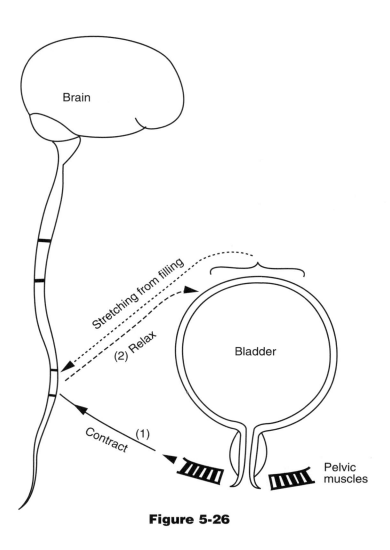

Figure 5-26

the intra-abdominal pressure pushing urine from the bladder.

If urge incontinence is a problem, (the sudden strong need to toilet before an individual can reach the bathroom), the bladder/detrusor muscle is contracting too frequently and at too great an intensity, thus over-powering the pelvic and urogenital diaphragm muscle support and urethral closure. A relatively large amount of urine is released before getting to the toilet.

If mixed incontinence is a problem there is a combination of stress and urge symptoms.

Constipation and Diarrhea

If constipation is a problem the pelvic muscles and sphincters have an increased resting tone that tends to hold the bowel movement in instead of relaxing and letting it out. The lower colon is not moving the feces through the rectum and anus effectively so too much water is being absorbed and the feces is becoming hard and rock-like.

If diarrhea is a problem the pelvic muscles and sphincters may have a decreased resting tone that allows the loose stool to exit before absorption of water is complete. The lower colon is moving the feces too rapidly through the colon so there is not enough time for water absorption to occur.

CHAPTER 6

What is the Beyond Kegels® Protocol?

Since the late 1940s Kegel exercises have been recommended for treating incontinence. Initially the individual was instructed to tighten and release the pelvic muscles as often as 300-500 times a day. Dr. Arnold Kegel named the exercises and used them to help his postpartum women who were leaking.

In the last 15 years, it has become clear that there is more involved in bladder and bowel health. New exercise protocols have evolved based on the historical information previously discussed and new perspectives on the anatomy and function of the urinary and pelvic muscle systems. Additional factors including lifestyle changes and nervous system balance are understood as important components of treatment.

The Beyond Kegels® Protocol is described in this chapter. This protocol is designed to prevent and treat bladder and bowel dysfunction including stress, urge and mixed urinary incontinence and constipation, diarrhea and fecal soiling. The Beyond Kegels® Protocol has five components that work together for bladder and bowel health.

The five components are:
1) Lifestyle Changes
2) Physiological Quieting®
3) Roll for Control® Exercises

4) Wonder W'edge™ Inversion
5) Modalities (optional)

Lifestyle Changes

Lifestyle changes are the foundation for bladder and bowel continence. It is important to return to a normal lifestyle routine of drinking, eating, physical, recreational and social activity.

The three most critical lifestyle changes are:
1) sleep,
2) nutrition including fluids, fruits and vegetables, and
3) walking.

Guidelines

Fluids: Six to eight 8-ounce glasses of non-caffeinated fluid a day is a general rule to follow; enough non-caffeinated fluid so an individual is toileting every 3-4 hours for 10-20 seconds of good stream flow and the urine is a light yellow color and without a strong odor.

Nutrition: Six to eight half-cup servings of fresh, raw or lightly cooked fruits and vegetables is a general rule to follow. Fruits and vegetables are essential for overall good health.

Constipation: The best fruit to eat when constipation is a problem is a fresh pear. Other good fruits to normalize a bowel movement are: peaches, plums, melons, berries and citrus fruit. Vegetables that are beneficial include dark green vegetables like broccoli, spinach, kale and beans.

Diarrhea: When diarrhea is a problem, fruits that stabilize and slow the digestive system include bananas and apples. Beneficial vegetables include potatoes, carrots, and peas.

Sleep: Eight to nine hours of sleep a night without getting up to toilet is a general rule to follow. When nighttime frequency or leaking is a problem stop drinking after dinner and lie down for 30 minutes before going to sleep, then get up to toilet. This helps to empty the bladder and allows a longer sleep without needing to toilet. Use protective pads and sleep through the night rather than get up just in case you might leak. If you wake up feeling the urge to toilet, practice Physiological Quieting® and fall back to sleep.

During pregnancy and after 65 years-of-age it is normal to get up once or twice a night. Getting up more than once a night may cause sleep deprivation and impact general health as well as overall bladder and bowel control.

Walking: Walking 30 minutes a day is a general rule to follow. Walking stimulates the smooth muscle of the bowel and bladder and strengthens the pelvic muscles that support the internal organs. An individual can start with 3-5 minutes at a time if he/she hasn't been walking. Two 15 minute walks or one 30 minute walk is optimal. Walking can be at an easy to moderate pace. It does not have to be aerobic or a cardiovascular tempo. More information on lifestyle changes is discussed in Chapter 7.

Physiological Quieting®

Physiological Quieting® techniques are another foundation for bladder and bowel continence. Physiological Quieting® techniques are used to re-balance the autonomic nervous system. The autonomic nervous system promotes efficient and effective bladder and bowel function. It controls pelvic muscle support and closure for the bladder and bowel. It controls the bladder and bowel irritability preventing overactive bladder and affecting irritable bowel syndrome (IBS).

The three most effective techniques to practice are:
1) diaphragmatic breathing,
2) handwarming, and
3) body-mind quieting.

Guidelines

Practice diaphragmatic breathing and handwarming when you wake in the morning and when you go to bed at night for 2-3 minutes. Then before each meal practice the same techniques for 30-60 seconds. More information on Physiological Quieting® is discussed in Chapter 8.

Roll for Control Exercises®

The Beyond Kegels® name came about after a significant number of individuals being treated for incontinence stated that Kegel exercises did not help them return to bladder and bowel health and control. The Beyond Kegels® Protocol was developed to improve the results from using Kegels exercises for bladder and bowel problems. Kegel exercises were very helpful for some people but many people found them difficult to understand and did not know if they were performing them correctly. Looking more completely into the structure and function of the pelvic muscles it was discovered that the support system for the bladder and bowel was more than the pelvic floor muscle. The support system was actually a combination of muscles extending through the lower pelvis and out to the leg bones (femurs). From this information the new Roll for Control® exercises, designed to stimulate action of the correct pelvic muscles combination, was developed. Our experience has covered 25 years specializing in the treatment of bladder and bowel health problems.

These exercises are easy to do. Children, the frail elderly even those who have experienced a stroke, multiple sclerosis, Parkinson's disease or dementia can do the exercises. They take less than 5 minutes twice a day and require no complicated equipment.

The Roll for Control® exercises include:
1) Relaxed awareness,
2) Heel and toe clicks,
3) Hip rolls, and
4) Standing Plies.

More information on Roll for Control Exercises is discussed in Chapter 9.

Wedge Inversion

Inversion on the Wonder W'edge™ is an important part of the Beyond Kegels® Protocol when there is any neurological or muscle damage from pregnancy, delivery, back pain, pelvic pain, surgical procedures, chronic constipation, chronic coughing, repetitive lifting, jumping or running, menopause or aging. When the pelvic diaphragm bowl descends for any reason the position of the sacrum and internal organs is altered.

Wonder W'edge™ inversion realigns the sacrum and internal organs so Roll for Control® exercises can be effective in bladder and bowel reeducation. The Wonder W'edge™ can be beneficial for both men and women. More information on Wonder W'edge™ inversion is discussed in Chapter 10.

Modalities

Biofeedback and electrical stimulation are two modalities used to treat bladder and bowel dysfunction. Chapter 12 discusses biofeedback in the use of bladder and bowel treatment.

CHAPTER 7

How Can I Alter My Personal And Social Environment?

An individual with leaking problems changes his/her behavior to accommodate the leaking. Changes may occur in:

1) what clothes are worn,
2) what location and supplies are used for sleep,
3) what activities outside the home are participated in,
4) what food and drink are consumed,
5) what friendships are maintained,
6) what intimate relationships are maintained or entered into,
7) what recreational or exercise activities are engaged in, and
8) what changes occur in self-concept and self-acceptance.

Clothing

An individual experiencing incontinence will often wear only dark or black pants or skirts to hide any wetness. Clothing has to be cleaned often, so washable clothing must be purchased. Taking a change of clothes wherever one goes is easier if they are wash-and-wear and lightweight so they can dry quickly and fit into a tote bag. Pants that are easily removed are important so leaking doesn't occur due to the delay caused by removing clothing.

Specialized, protective, reusable underpants are often worn in conjunction with incontinence pads. Other times, disposable briefs with absorbent pads are helpful. Some individuals use toweling, toilet paper, or sanitary pads in regular underpants to absorb leaks.

Nighttime Sleep
Some individuals have leaking problems at night. Various means of protection are used including an absorbent bed pad, towels placed on the bed, and specialized underpants and pads.

At times individuals are getting up to toilet from several times a night to hourly. Sleep is severely disrupted. Physiological Quieting® at bedtime and when the individual awakens in the night is helpful for this problem. It is important to use a pad at night and sleep through the night in most cases.

When leaking at night is prevalent, some individuals report moving from sleeping with a partner to sleeping alone until the problem diminishes. It is important to communicate with a partner about feelings and facts as well as listening to his/her needs before this change is made.

Food and Drink
One of the most common comments heard when someone has a leaking problem is "I quit drinking much so I

won't leak." Decreasing the liquid intake decreases the bladder size because the bladder stretches or shrinks depending on how much fluid is present. As the bladder shrinks from less and less fluid being ingested, the brain is told it is "full" more frequently and the brain then tells the bladder to empty the urine more frequently. The result can be toileting routines that are every 30-60 minutes instead of the normal routine of every 3-4 hours. Less fluid also concentrates the urine. The bladder wall is more likely to be irritated by the concentrated urine which can set off bladder contractions. The common misconception is that less fluid decreases leaking. The reality is that less fluid increases frequency of urination and bladder irritability which often leads to more leaking. Therefore, drinking adequate fluid, six to eight, 8-ounce glasses, is recommended.

Alcoholic beverages are not recommended. They alter the nervous system and can be a bladder irritant. It is therefore important for individuals experiencing incontinence to eliminate alcoholic beverages from their diet.

Caffeine is a highly irritating substance to the nervous system controlling the bladder and bowel. The residue it leaves in urine is an irritant to the bladder wall. Eliminating caffeine, including coffee, sodas, teas, and chocolate, may decrease or eliminate incontinence.

Some individuals will use food as an emotional support or to cover up feelings when there is embarrassment and loss of control stemming from incontinence. The increased food intake leads to weight gain. Even a five-pound weight gain can increase incontinence. The types of food eaten can affect incontinence too. Increasing the intake of fruits and vegetables will increase fluids and vitamin/mineral levels while decreasing overall calorie intake. Eating unprocessed foods avoids chemicals that may be irritating to the bladder or nervous system. Acidic fruits and vegetables can be irritating to the bladder. Artificial sweeteners, colors and flavors may also be irritating to the bladder.

Friendships

Isolation can be a problem when the individual with incontinence is embarrassed by urine loss and is fearful someone will notice an offensive odor, a wet spot on his/her clothes, the bulge of pads used, or the frequency with which she/he uses the toilet. The ultimate fear is of a major accident when with friends or in public. It is important not to let these fears interfere with social activity. Outings with friends and family are essential to a happy, healthy life. Plan ahead, wear comfortable clothing, bring a change of clothing, wear pads or protective undergarments. Do whatever is necessary to be with friends and family.

It is important to tell friends about a leaking problem in a brief but informative way. "My bladder is malfunctioning so I need to use the bathroom frequently," is what Mona told her friend when they went shopping. Speaking up the first time is the hardest. It is important to maintain friendships since isolation leads to depression in even the healthiest person. Linda shared how she viewed her problem: "Incontinence is no different than poor eyesight. I use pads and do exercises for my leaking problem just like I wear glasses to improve my eyesight. Then I get on with my life, love, and happiness."

Intimate Relationships

Intimate relationships are an important consideration when dealing with incontinence. The partner in an established relationship needs to be informed about the problem and possible solutions in order to maintain physical and emotional closeness. Sharing feelings, both positive and negative, helps both partners continue the relationship. Try alternately listening to each other after asking the questions, "How do you feel about this leaking?" "What are the aspects you are comfortable with?" "What parts make you feel uncomfortable?" "What are your needs and how can I be involved?"

Expanding the definition of intimacy can be helpful in any relationship. Sometimes leaking occurs during intercourse. Using a towel or having intercourse in the hot tub or shower are options. Changing positions from the missionary position to side-lying or all-fours with rear entry may put less pressure on the bladder.

Intimacy also includes physical hugging, caresses, and kissing; it can be verbal expressions of caring, it can be music, it can be movement in the form of dance, it can be fragrances in the environment, it can be the written word-25 reasons I love you, or a daily special note at the breakfast table. Intimacy can take many forms if we open our minds and hearts to love, and it should never be disrupted by a little leaking.

Recreational Activities

Maintaining an active and enjoyable lifestyle is an important aspect in treating incontinence. Physical exercise is vital to physical and emotional health. Physical exercise increases the endorphins-chemicals that elevate mood and are often called the "good humor hormones." Physical activity increases metabolism to help maintain weight control. Physical activity tones and strengthens muscles throughout the body. Too often, physical exercise is eliminated in an attempt not to leak. As 40-year-old Judy commented, "When I jogged or skied I leaked, so I quit jogging and skiing." Rather than quitting a favorite activity, it is important to make adaptations in order to continue the activity without embarrassment. Use a superabsorbant pad. Take breaks that allow time for toileting and plan ahead where the toilets will be. Bring extra clothing in case an accident occurs.

Incontinence can also be the impetus to try new activities. Instead of jogging Judy tried rollerblading and bowling. She met new friends participating in these new activities and widened her perspective on what can be fun to do in her free time.

Self Concept and Self Esteem

Feelings of shame and embarrassment about leaking often become generalized to the whole person negatively affecting self-esteem. Common symptoms include sadness, lack of energy, change in eating habits, and sleep disruption. Identifying with infantile or aging behavior rather than healthy, active adult behavior may be experienced. Confidence can turn to feelings of vulnerability, frustration, and anger. Examples of negative self-talk include, "I smell repulsive," "I can't go anywhere if the toilet isn't close by," "I act like a baby and treat myself like one," "If I were a stronger person, I could control this leaking," "My body is going downhill, losing control, and soon I'll be ready for a nursing home or the graveyard."

Active coping strategies are essential to positive self-esteem and self-concept. These include:

1) Admit and identify the leaking problem.
2) Assertively gather information about your specific problem. Consult books, physicians, and support groups.
3) Consider all possible solutions before making educated decisions.
4) Develop and practice positive self-statements.
5) Practice self-reliance while changing life style habits that will facilitate being dry.

Self Talk - Positive Self Statements

The mind is always saying something positive, negative, or neutral as an individual goes through the day. Even while sleeping at night there are thoughts and dreams. Self talk can be helpful or hurtful in relation to incontinence symptoms and an individual's accomplishments. To develop an awareness of what self talk is like, for one or two days pause four or five times during the day and jot down what thoughts are present at that time in relation to what you are doing and how you are feeling. Are they primarily positive or negative thoughts? Are there repetitive thoughts? Now take the positive thoughts and repeat them throughout the day. Pair the positive self statement with some event that occurs frequently in the day. If there is negative self talk, substitute positive statements for the negative thoughts.

Examples of positive self statements are:
1) I am an active energetic adult who can solve a leaking problem.
2) I am trying, I am doing the best I can.
3) I deserve to be healthy and active, I am healthy and active.
4) I deserve to sleep through the night and be dry. I sleep through the night and am dry.
5) I can make adaptations and be active.

For some individuals, positive self statements seem like lies or half truths. If that occurs, put "I am trying" or "I am beginning to" in front of the statement. Remember every thought stimulates biomechanical and electrical events in the brain and gut which then flow to every cell of the body and affect all other body and mind functions.

Getting Started and Keeping Track of Changes

To begin life style changes, pick two or three of the ideas just discussed and begin to implement them. For instance, the first week:

1) Eliminate all caffeine and alcohol, including colas, coffee, and chocolate.
2) Drink six to eight glasses of fluid a day to maintain the size of the bladder and also to dilute the concentration of urine.
3) Do some fun and purposeless activity every day. Thirty minutes of walking, swimming, or biking daily will help to improve pelvic muscle function and maintain overall good health.
4) Eat a fresh pear or peach a day if constipation is a problem.

To see progress, keep a daily journal. Record the glasses of fluid consumed, the caffeine consumed, the activity participated in, and the amount of time spent on the activity.

CHAPTER 8

How Can I Balance My Body? Physiological Quieting® (PQ)

Individuals experiencing incontinence are often experiencing excessive arousal and imbalance of the autonomic nervous system. One result is an overactive bladder (detrusor) muscle that tells the brain it needs to empty too frequently. Another result is elevated pelvic muscle resting tone which can lead to constipation, poor urine flow or pain.

The bladder muscle contracts or relaxes depending on how full the bladder is perceived to be by the brain. The autonomic nervous system is the telephone system that sends messages between the brain and the bladder telling the bladder to contract or relax. If the telephone system that operates the bladder thinks that the bladder is full, the message system tells the bladder to contract. That message should be heard every 3-4 hours to prompt you to go to the toilet. Sometimes the message system gets confused as to how much urine is really in the bladder. There may be very little urine in the bladder yet the message system tells the bladder to contract and you feel the need to go to the toilet. Frequent toileting can disrupt your life and cause you to be afraid to go places and plan activities. You can stop the too frequent feeling of urges that tell you to go to the bathroom. Physiological Quieting® techniques can rebalance the autonomic nervous system and train the bladder and bowel to relax until it is full.

Physiological Quieting® is often overlooked or ignored while you do the exercises. In fact many people try to avoid doing it altogether because it seems strange and unfamiliar compared to doing exercises. "Believe me it works!!" Kari exclaims after she used the CD for a week. "Before I didn't understand exactly how it could help and I wasn't sure my partner would want to hear it as we went to sleep. Now he asks where it is if I don't put it on." Joe states "It relaxes me, it gives my whole body a health bonus while it returns my bladder to its calm and relaxed state." "I used to have urges almost every hour and had to run to the bathroom. Now after several weeks of listening to the Physiological Quieting® CD at night my uncontrollable bladder urges are gone." Mary commented.

It is possible to listen to the CD privately during the day or by using earphones, but sharing it with some-one else can be helpful to both of you. Even children can benefit from Physiological Quieting® in the PQ for Kids CD. The Physiological Quieting® techniques help you tune into your muscles as you release them and help you condition the message system from the brain to the bladder and bowel so they function at their opti-mum levels.

Learning the Physiological Quieting® techniques of breathing, handwarming and body-mind quieting will erase the confusion in the message system and allow the bladder and bowel to relax while filling and the pelvic muscles to support the bladder and bowel in their optimal position.

Here is how it works. The telephone system that communicates with your bladder also communicates with all other muscles of the body. Learning Physiological Quieting® teaches the body's telephone messages to slow down and be quieter. At the same time Physiological Quieting® tells the bladder muscle to slow down and be quieter because the messages from the brain to the bladder along the telephone lines are slower and quieter. When you learn the Physiological Quieting® techniques of diaphragmatic breathing, handwarming, and body-mind quieting specific muscles in your body release and relax. At the same time your breathing slows and your bladder quiets because there is a spill over effect. All parts of your body are connected to all other parts. Remember the song "The leg bone is connected to the ankle bone. The ankle bone is connected to the foot bone." Even muscles you are not aware of being able to control, like the bladder, are affected when you change muscles you can control. Listen to the Physiological Quieting® CD nightly and practice handwarming and diaphragmatic breathing hourly for 30 seconds. In 4-6 weeks your autonomic nervous system will be more balanced, your bladder frequency and urgency decreased and your bowel more regular.

Physiological Quieting® includes:
1) Diaphragmatic Breathing
2) Handwarming
3) Body/Mind Quieting

Diaphragmatic Breathing

The diaphragm is a large sheet-like muscle that rests in a dome shape in the chest cavity. As you inhale the dome flattens and pulls down to the bottom of the rib-cage. During exhale the diaphragm moves back to the dome shape. When breathing correctly, the shoulder and chest areas remain quiet, the jaw is relaxed, and the teeth are separated. The abdominal wall expands to accommodate the downward pressure on the internal organs.

To practice:

"Inhale, let my abdomen rise. Exhale, let my abdomen fall. Quiet shoulders, quiet chest. Jaw released, teeth apart, tongue off the roof of my mouth."

There is equal time for inhale and exhale. Inhale through the nose, exhale through the mouth or nose.

Practice diaphragmatic breathing initially in a reclined position, then in sitting and standing. Practice 4-5 diaphragmatic breaths every hour during the day if you experience overactive bladder, irritable bowel syndrome or pelvic pain. Practice 3-4 times a day if you experience stress incontinence or constipation.

Hand Warming

Hand warming is a technique that rebalances the autonomic nervous system to normalize bladder and bowel function. The autonomic nervous system controls blood vessel dilation to increase blood volume to body parts including your hands and fingers while at the same time it normalizes your bladder and bowel function. Mental imaging and frequently repeated thoughts transfer information to nerve activity that balances the sympathetic nervous system with the parasympathetic. This autonomic nervous system balance in turn inhibits bladder contractions and increases blood flow to the hands.

To accomplish this:

1) Focus on your hands and say to yourself, "My hands are warmer and warmer, warmth is flowing into my hands, warmer and warmer."

2) Imagine the warmest color and surround your hands and wrists with that color. Let that color flow into your hands, deep into the fingers, palms, wrists while they get warmer and warmer.

3) Feel the warmest, safest place your hands can be: Holding a warm cup of hot chocolate, holding your hands over a camp fire or radiator, or slipping your hands and feet into the hot sand of a beach on a summer day.

To accomplish a resetting of the autonomic nervous system, i.e. to slow the high idle, it is necessary to frequently practice the techniques to quiet the system for short periods. The instructions are: "Practice hourly for 30-60 seconds."

Body/Mind Quieting

Excessive bladder and pelvic muscle resting tone and increased activity level of bladder and bowel contractions can be decreased through Physiological Quieting®.

Find a quiet, warm room with a chair or bed that gives complete support from your head to your feet. Use pillows for support of your neck, low back, arms, and knees where needed for comfort.

Then,

1) Focus on your breathing, feel the pattern of breathing, let your abdomen rise with inhale, fall with exhale.
2) Feel the support of the bed or chair and release into that support from the top of your head to the tips of your toes.
3) Focus on your face and neck. Notice where there is any tension or tightness, where there is quiet, calmness in each part of your face and neck. Then, say to yourself 3-4 times, "My face and neck muscles are quiet and calm, my face and neck muscles are calmer and calmer."
4) Proceed from head to toe in the same manner, focusing on each body part as you did the face and neck.
5) Focus again on diaphragmatic breathing.

Listen to the Physiological Quieting® CD or practice on your own nightly for 4-6 weeks.

CHAPTER 9

What Exercises Can Help?
Roll for Control® Exercises

In the 1970s Kegel exercises were focused on women during pregnancy and postpartum. They were taught in childbirth education classes when the instruction was to tighten and release the pelvic muscles 100-200 times a day. The instructor would say, "Every time you go to the refrigerator or are at a stop sign, do 10. " By the late 1980s, Kegel exercises included quick contractions and ten-second-hold contractions practiced 20 minutes twice a day.

Originally little thought was given to other muscles contracting when the pelvic muscles tightened. The instruction was to tighten as much as possible. It was common for abdominal and gluteal muscles to tighten as much as the pelvic muscles. By the early 1990s the exercise prescription was to inhibit or prevent the abdominal and gluteal muscles tightening with pelvic muscle contraction. The instruction was to "keep your tummy and buttocks quiet and relaxed while you lift your pelvic muscles up and in." During this same period the concept of breath control with pelvic muscle contractions became important. Since breath-holding increases intra-abdominal pressure, bladder pressure, and leaking, the instructions were to "keep breathing while you tighten the pelvic muscles."

In the early 1990s, the typical exercise program included the following:

- quick contract and release of the pelvic muscles,
- ten second hold, ten second rest of the pelvic muscles,
- relaxed abdominal and buttocks muscles during pelvic muscle contraction, and
- breath control during pelvic muscle contractions for
- 20 minute practice sessions twice a day.

These exercises helped some individuals progress from constant or intermittent leaking to being dry in 6-12 weeks. They were primarily recommended for stress incontinence problems, relatively small leaks when coughing, running, jumping, lifting, or bending. Urge incontinence was not thought to be treatable through exercise.

In the last 15 years, a new exercise protocol has evolved based on the historical information previously discussed and new perspectives on the anatomy and function of the urinary, bowel and pelvic muscle systems.

The Roll for Control® exercises are described in this chapter. This exercise series is designed to prevent and treat bladder and bowel dysfunction including diagnoses of stress, urge and mixed urinary incontinence, constipation, fecal soiling and diarrhea.

Before starting the exercises, there are several training principles important to remember in any bladder and bowel exercise program.

Training Principles of Exercise

1) Overload Principle
2) Specificity Principle
3) Maintenance Principle
4) Reversibility Principle
5) Motor Control Principle

The overload principle states that for pelvic muscles to strengthen, they must be pushed to the limit and just a little beyond. If over-exercised, the muscles fatigue and cannot function, so other muscles must try to compensate. The abdominal and gluteal muscles will become more active when the pelvic muscles fatigue. If the muscles are under-exercised, they are not challenged to increase in strength, endurance, or speed. Their length and resting tone remain the same.

The specificity principle states that the pelvic muscles are composed of fast twitch and slow twitch fibers roughly in a 35%:65% ratio. Some muscles have a combination of fast and slow twitch components. Fast twitch fibers improve in speed and strength with quick explosive contractions, while slow twitch fibers strengthen and gain optimal resting length and tone with longer "hold" contractions, (10 second hold, 10 second rest periods rather than 1-2 second hold and rest periods). Fast twitch fibers fatigue quickly, so 5-10 repetitions is adequate. Slow twitch fibers are designed for endurance and postural tone, so more repetitions are possible before fatigue occurs.

The maintenance principle describes exercising for continence as a lifelong endeavor. Once a person is dry, pelvic muscle function is maintained by integrating exercise into daily activities. The pelvic muscles are no different than leg, heart, or lung muscles. They need exercise to remain healthy.

The reversibility principle states that if, after an individual exercises and becomes dry or continent, she/he then quits exercising, it will take three times as long for the pelvic muscles to return to their original strength as it did to reach the continent level of strength. For example, if it took three months to exercise to the point of continence, it will take nine months of not exercising to decrease tone and strength of the pelvic muscles to again experience leaking.

The motor control principle states that exercise designed to improve functional activity involves exercising the muscles as a group using submaximal contraction of muscles, equal work and rest periods and low number of repetitions done several times a day.

A consistent and effective exercise program is an important commitment. The Roll for Control® exercise series is developed in four levels for that purpose. The levels are designed to progress in body awareness, muscle fiber type, and level of exercise difficulty. Begin with Level One, even though it seems very simple, and progress through the four levels sequentially in one to two weeks. Level One, Relaxed Awareness of the Pelvic Muscles, sets the stage for integrating body awareness and breathing with isolated pelvic muscle exercises. Level Two facilitates improved function of the slow twitch, postural fibers of the pelvic diaphragm/levator ani, obturator internus, and adductor muscles. Level Three strengthens the fast twitch fibers primarily of the urogenital diaphragm muscles. Level Four Standing Plié, facilitates the pelvic rotator cuff action in functional activities.

Exercise length and duration are determined by the results of the initial evaluation of pelvic muscle function. In general, start by exercising as follows:

First Week: 5-10 repetitions, 3 times a day.

Second Week: 10 repetitions, 3 times a day.

Level One
Relaxed Awareness of the Pelvic Muscles

The first level is relaxed awareness of the pelvic muscles. (Fig. 9-1) In a comfortable, supported position reclining on a bed or semi-sitting or sitting in a chair, concentrate on how the chair or bed feels from your head to your feet. Feel that support and relax into that support, letting go into the support more and more through your head and neck, shoulders and back, arms and hands; let your hips and legs sink into the support, let your ankles and feet relax and release into the bed or the chair.

Now notice your breathing. Notice the natural rhythm of your breathing. Inhale.....Exhale...... Think,

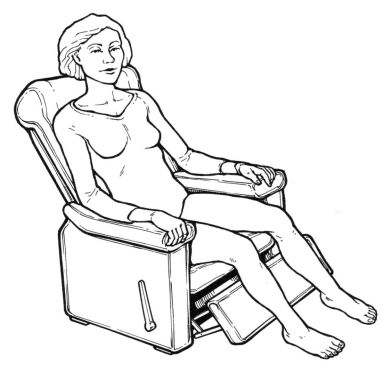

Figure 9-1

"Quiet shoulders, quiet chest." Let your stomach rise with your inhale, fall with your exhale. Now notice your stomach muscles and your buttocks muscles. Let them be relaxed and totally released. Connect your mind to the hammock of muscles that forms the base of the pelvis, the hammock of muscles running from the symphysis pubis in the front to the tail bone or coccyx in the back. Maintaining your breathing rhythm, gently tighten this hammock of muscles, gently lift up and in to tighten, then release, gently and easily. Try again, tighten and release as if to stop urinating, maintaining your breathing, keeping your stomach and buttocks relaxed. Do 3 or 4 of these gentle contractions, keeping your mind connected to the hammock of muscles.

Practice this exercise for 30-60 seconds at the beginning and ending of each exercise session.

Level Two-A
Assisted Pelvic Muscle Tightening
Using Adductors/Inner Thigh Muscles

For this exercise you will be using a Roll for Control® Ball, a 7"-9" soft ball. Sit or recline with your feet hip width apart. Place the ball between your legs just above the knees. Now roll your knees in against the ball. Hold for a count of 10. Now relax and release your knees for a count of 10. (Fig. 9-2) Remember, as you do this exercise, to maintain your breathing rhythm, and tighten just the muscles of your inner thighs. The pelvic floor tightens automatically when your knees roll in. When this is easy, rotate your toes together, pivoting on your heels at the same time you roll your knees in squeezing the ball. Hold for a count of 10. Release and relax for a count of 10. The muscles of your abdomen and buttocks should remain relaxed and loose.

Repeat this exercise 2-3 times a day for 5-10 repetitions. Continue until this exercise is easy to do. This will often take 5-7 days. Then add the next exercise.

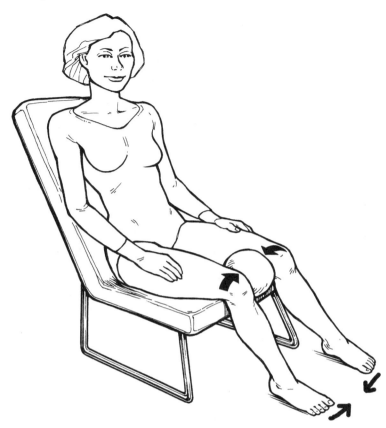

Figure 9-2

Level Two-O
Assisted Pelvic Muscle Tightening
Using Obturator Internus Muscles/Hip Rotators

This level of exercise facilitates action of pelvic dia-phragm/ levator ani muscles by using the obturator internus muscle. (Fig. 9-3) In this exercise, the Roll for Control® band, an elastic band 1"-2" wide, is secured around the legs just above the knees while squeezing your thighs together. Your heels are touching. Now roll your knees out 3-4 inches against the elastic band. Hold the position while you count to 10 slowly. Then relax the muscles completely and return to the neutral position for a count of 10. Maintaining your breathing rhythm, try this exercise again. When this is easy, rotate your toes away from each other pivoting on your heels at the same time you roll your knees out against the band. Remember that rolling your knees out while using the small hip rotator muscles (the obturator internus), assists the pelvic diaphragm/levator ani muscles in support and stabilization of the bladder, urethra, and bowel, rectum and anus.

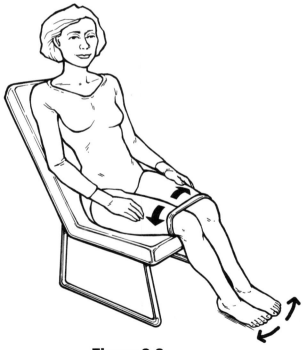

Figure 9-3

Repeat this exercise 2-3 times a day for 5-10 repetitions. When it is easy to do, add the next exercise in this level.

Level Two-A&O
Combining Inner and Outer Thigh Muscles
Adductor and obturator muscle assist-exercises are combined into one when they are easy to do. This exercise then becomes the only exercise done for level two.

Roll your knees in against the Roll for Control® ball, and pivot your toes toward each other, holding for a count of 10. Then release and relax for a count of 10.

Now roll your knees out against the Roll for Control® band, and pivot your toes away from each other, holding for a count of 10. Then relax and release for a count of 10. Repeat this exercise 5-10 times. (Fig. 9-4)

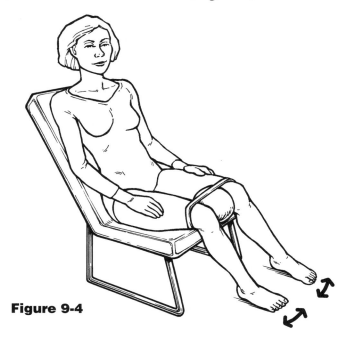

Figure 9-4

103

Level Three
Heel Clicks and Toe Clicks

The exercise in this level improves the strength and function of the fast acting fibers primarily of the urogenital diaphragm and external sphincter muscles. These fibers are important for prevention of leaking during coughing and sneezing or any sudden increase in intra-abdominal pressure.

To perform this exercise, focus on your breathing rhythm maintaining that breathing rhythm while you perform the exercises. Sit with your feet hip width apart. Pivoting on your toes and forefeet squeeze your heels together for a count of two. Then return to the neutral position and rest for a count of two. Repeat this five times.

Next, pivot on your heels and squeeze your toes together for a count of two. Then return to the neutral position and rest for a count of two. Repeat this five times.

As you squeeze your heels or toes together think or say, "Squeeze.....and release." (Fig. 9-5) It is as important to release completely and quickly as it is to tighten forcefully.

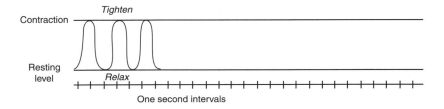

Figure 9-5

104

Level Four
Standing Plié Small Knee Bends

Many of our daily activities involve standing and most leaking occurs during standing activities, so the pelvic muscles must function effectively in this position to prevent leaking.

Stand with your feet hip-width apart with your feet turned outward. Now do a small plié, bending the knees 2"-3" for a slow count of 5 as you rotate your knees over your toes. Then return slowly to the upright

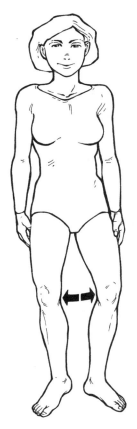

position for a slow count of 5 as you rotate your knees toward the midline. The knee-bend position with the feet pointed outward activates the obturator internus muscle in combination with the pelvic diaphragm/levator ani muscles. Inhale as you bend your knees and exhale as you straighten your knees. (Fig. 9-6)

Repeat this exercise 5 times initially. Gradually increase to 10 repetitions during an exercise session. This is a good exercise to do while standing brushing your teeth or in line at the grocery store or movies.

Figure 9-6

105

CHAPTER 10

How Do I Use Wonder W'edge™ Inversion?

Inversion on the Wonder W'edge™ is an important part of the Beyond Kegels® Protocol if there is any neurological or muscle damage from back pain, pregnancy, delivery, surgical procedures, chronic constipation, chronic coughing, repetitive lifting, jumping or running, menopause or aging. When the pelvic diaphragm bowl descends for any reason the position of the sacrum and internal organs is altered. Wonder W'edge™ inversion realigns the sacrum and internal organs so Roll for Control® exercises can be effective in bladder and bowel reeducation. The Wonder W'edge™ can be beneficial for both men and women. (Fig. 10-1)

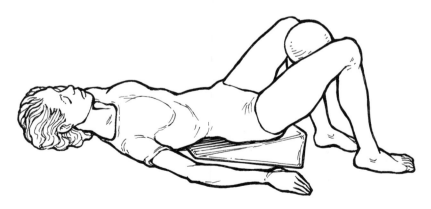

Figure 10-1

Pelvic Relaxation Syndrome

As the pelvic diaphragm descends the bladder, bowel and uterus descend lower in the pelvis, become less stable and exhibit impaired function. The urethral closure mechanisms becomes less effective, the anorectal angle and external sphincter in the bowel changes. This descent of organs is termed pelvic relaxation syndrome and includes cystocele, uterine prolapse, enterocele and rectocele.

As pelvic muscles and organs descend they pull the sacrum out of alignment with the pelvis. Sacroiliac joint dysfunction and back pain is reported. As the pelvic muscles and organs descend they pull on sacral nerves that innervate the pelvic muscles and descend down the legs to the feet. Leg pain and foot pain is another frequent complaint with pelvic muscle and internal organ descent. Wonder W'edge™ inversion realigns the internal organs within the pelvis and repositions them so they are again appropriately supported by the sacrum. The Wonder W'edge™ aligns the sacrum into a more stable position relieving stress on the lower lumbar and sacral nerves. Then when Roll for Control® exercises are done on the Wonder W'edge™ the pelvic diaphragm is lifted into a correct supportive position for the internal organs and sacrum.

When Roll for Control® exercises are done without first correcting pelvic diaphragm and internal organ descent the muscles squeeze around the descended organs and may even squeeze them lower into the pelvis. Realigning internal organs and pelvic muscle using inversion can relieve symptoms of back, leg and foot pain. It may also improve your ability to stand for longer periods of time.

There are some individuals with cardiac, pulmonary and cervical problems that cannot use the Wonder W'edge™ for inversion. Each individual should find a comfortable position on the Wonder W'edge™ by adjusting his/her hips and back on the wedge with the neck and head in a neutral position.

Alignment on the Wonder W'edge™: To align for inversion on the Wonder W'edge place the wedge on the floor or on your bed. Sit next to it and then lift your hips onto the high end of the wedge while your shoulders and head are off the wedge. Find a position that is comfortable with your hips as high on the wedge as possible. Your feet can be resting flat on the floor or on the wall or on a large therapeutic ball.

Diaphragmatic Breathing on the Wonder W'edge™: Once you are comfortable on the wedge the next step is to practice 6-8 diaphragmatic breaths. First notice your natural breathing pattern. Notice your inhale and exhale. Then notice where your breathing occurs. Is there movement in your abdomen, chest, shoulders, back, neck or jaw? Now think, "Inhale, let my abdomen rise. Exhale, let my abdomen fall". Then as you inhale and exhale think, "Quiet shoulders, quiet chest". Next as you inhale and exhale think, "Jaw released, teeth apart, tongue at the bottom of my mouth". Let your breath come naturally thinking, "Slow and low, my breathing is slow and low".

Roll for Control® Exercises on the Wonder W'edge™: Once you are comfortable on the wedge and have practiced diaphragmatic breathing you can add Roll for Control® Exercises. If the Wonder W'edge™ is helpful, practice your exercises on the wedge at least once a day.

CHAPTER 11

How Do Treatments Differ for: Stress and Urge Incontinence? Constipation and Diarrhea?

Beyond Kegels® Protocol Based on Type of Bladder and Bowel Dysfunction

Beyond Kegels® Protocol differs for each type of dysfunction. They include:

1) Stress Urinary Incontinence Protocol
2) Urge Urinary Incontinence Protocol
3) Mixed Urinary Incontinence Protocol
4) Constipation Protocol
5) Diarrhea Protocol

Stress Incontinence Protocol includes:

1) Lifestyle Changes including sleep, nutrition and walking.
2) Physiological Quieting® using the CD at night when going to sleep and practicing short periods of breathing and handwarming 3-4 times during the day.
3) Level One Exercise. Inhibit excessive resting tone of the pelvic and abdominal muscles through Physiological Quieting®. This decreases excessive intra-abdominal pressure and assists the pelvic muscles in resting when appropriate and contracting quickly and intensely when needed.

4) Level Two and Four Exercises. Strengthen slow twitch fibers of the pelvic diaphragm/levator ani and obturator internus muscles to obtain optimal alignment of the bladder, bladder neck and urethra.
5) Level Three Exercise. Strengthen fast twitch fibers of the urogenital diaphragm muscles for quick response when coughing, sneezing or physical activity that increases intra-abdominal pressure suddenly.

Urge Incontinence Protocol includes:
1) Lifestyle Changes including sleep, nutrition and walking.
2) Physiological Quieting® techniques using the CD at night when going to sleep and practicing diaphragmatic breathing and handwarming 30 seconds hourly.
3) Level One Exercise. This exercise improves the mind's connection to the bladder and pelvic muscle region. This exercise quiets the overactive bladder by decreasing intra-abdominal pressure, i.e., relaxed, toned abdominal muscles. It enables the individual to isolate pelvic muscle activity from abdominal and gluteal muscle contractions.
4) Level Three Exercise. Strengthen fast twitch fibers of the urogenital diaphragm muscles for quieting the overactive bladder muscle.
5) Level Two and Four Exercises. Strengthen the pelvic diaphragm/levator ani muscles to obtain optimum position of bladder, bladder neck and urethra.

Mixed Incontinence Protocol includes:

The combination of exercises for stress and urge incontinence is effective for mixed incontinence symptoms.

Constipation Protocol includes:

1) Lifestyle Changes including sleep, nutrition and walking. Changes in nutrition are often important in changing the consistency of the bowel movement. Adding foods that move through the intestines more quickly is important. Fruits include fresh pear, peach, plum, orange and grapefruit, melon, and berries. Vegetables include fresh spinach, kale, broccoli and beans. Adequate fluid is important, at least 4-8 glasses of fluid that is non-caffeinated.

2) Physiological Quieting® techniques using the CD at night when going to sleep and practicing diaphragmatic breathing and handwarming 3-4 times a day normalizes bowel tone and facilitates normal peristalsis.

3) Level One Exercise. Inhibit excessive resting tone of the pelvic and abdominal muscles through Physiological Quieting®. This decreases excessive intra-abdominal pressure and assists the pelvic muscles in resting when appropriate and contracting quickly and intensely when needed.

4) Level Two and Four Exercises. Strengthen slow twitch fibers of the pelvic diaphragm, adductors, and obturator internus muscles to obtain optimal alignment of the anus, rectum and anorectal angle.

5) Level Three Exercise. Strengthen fast twitch fibers of the anal sphincter muscles for quick response

when coughing, sneezing or physical activity that increases intra-abdominal pressure suddenly.

Diarrhea Protocol includes:

1) Lifestyle Changes including sleep, nutrition and walking. Changes in nutrition are often important in changing the consistency of the bowel movement. Adding foods that move through the intestines more slowly is important. Fruits include banana and apple or applesauce. Vegetables include white potatoes, rice, and pasta. Limit fluid if you are drinking a lot and avoid caffeine.

2) Physiological Quieting® techniques using the CD at night when going to sleep and practicing diaphragmatic breathing and handwarming 3-4 times a day normalizes the bowel peristalsis.

3) Level One Exercise. Inhibit excessive resting tone of the pelvic and abdominal muscles. This decreases excessive intra-abdominal pressure and assists the pelvic muscles in resting when appropriate and contracting quickly and intensely when needed.

4) Level Two and Four Exercises. Strengthen slow twitch fibers of the pelvic diaphragm, adductor, and obturator internus muscles to obtain optimal alignment of the rectum, anus & anorectal angle.

5) Level Three Exercise. Strengthen fast twitch fibers of the anal sphincter muscles for quick response when coughing, sneezing or physical activity that increases intra-abdominal pressure suddenly.

CHAPTER 12

How Can Biofeedback Help With Exercise For Incontinence?

Biofeedback:

How can it help with exercises for incontinence?

By taking the guesswork out of doing a movement that can't be seen.

Biofeedback measures and displays information occurring within the body, information about muscle tension (electrical activity of muscles), circulation and breathing patterns. This is information a person normally does not perceive, information at an unconscious level. Biofeedback enables an individual to become aware of these processes at a conscious level.

Biofeedback is like a mirror: it shows the individual what the muscles are doing inside the body as they contract and relax. There are many muscles in the region that may be tightened when attempting to tighten the pelvic and urogenital diaphragm muscles. Biofeedback is a mirror that lets an individual separate one muscle group from the others. Just like the visual image in the mirror, biofeedback brings the image of muscle action to a screen so changes can be made quickly and accurately. If a woman wants to part her hair on the other side or put lipstick on her lips she uses the mirror to tell her first that it needs to be done and second that the changes she made are what she wants and where she wants them. Biofeedback tells the individual what the pelvic muscles are doing in isolation from other muscles, and it shows changes in the action of the muscles immediately and accurately as the individual tightens or relaxes them.

Biofeedback was first used to treat incontinence by Arnold Kegel, M.D., in the 1940s. He used a perineometer which measured pressure in the vaginal canal. The pressure increased when the pelvic muscles tightened and decreased when they relaxed. The original Kegel exercises were done using this method.

Today, biofeedback for urinary incontinence is a training method that gives quick, accurate information to the individual about pelvic muscle tightness and muscle relaxation via a monitor or a repetitive sound or a blinking light display. This immediate information improves learning new skills, such as tightening and relaxing pelvic muscles, because it helps the individual make immediate adjustments in the muscle activity depending on the desired action. Small sensors, connected to the biofeedback equipment, pick up and accurately measure activity of the pelvic muscles. This information is instantly transferred to the screen or display for the individual to see or hear.

Biofeedback for incontinence can provide information about the pelvic and urogential diaphragm muscles and the anal sphincter. Pelvic muscle activity can be monitored directly through sensors recording the electrical activity at the nerve-muscle connection. This is called electromyography (EMG). Surface sensors are applied to the skin surface over the muscle group. Internal vaginal or anal sensors are self-inserted in the vagina or anus to pick up pelvic muscle activity closer to the muscle surface. Surface sensors can also monitor abdominal, gluteal, adductor, and breathing diaphragm muscles.

Sensors pick up even slight contractions of the pelvic and urogential diaphragm muscles when the individual tries to tighten them and the intensity and pattern of the contraction is visible immediately on the biofeedback display. A stronger contraction of the same muscles can be attempted and the observable difference between the two pictures is reinforcement for improved function of the pelvic muscles with each new contraction. As Martha said during her first biofeedback session, "Oh, so this is how it is supposed to feel when I do the exercise! I thought I was doing it right before but I wasn't using the right muscles." The guesswork is taken out of doing a movement that cannot be seen. The feel of the exercise is paired with the objective picture on the screen so changes are made more quickly. Problems with both stress and urge incontinence can be helped with this type of biofeedback.

The bladder (detrusor) and bowel muscles are not under our voluntary control, but an individual can learn to quiet their tone through biofeedback that indirectly monitors the autonomic or "automatic" nervous system that controls the bladder. Although it is not possible to directly control the bladder or bowel, Physiological

Quieting® will normalize the bladder and bowel since they receive their innervation from the autonomic nervous system. This nervous system controls breathing rate and circulation. If an individual learns to slow the breathing rate or warm the hands by increasing blood flow to the hands, there is a generalized effect to the bladder and bowel. The bladder quiets so the frequent urge to urinate decreases as the individual's breathing slows and hands warm. Sensors that pick up hand temperature tell the individual if the circulation is improving by showing the rising temperature on a monitor (for example from 86.5° to 88.7°). Sensors that measure movement of the diaphragm tell the individual how many breaths per minute occur and how effectively the diaphragm is being used by showing diaphragm muscle activity on the monitor. Problems with urge incontinence, an unstable bladder, can be helped using this type of biofeedback.

Biofeedback can be used at home as well as in the clinic. Small home units are available that have their own small screens or attach to the monitor. The sensors are easy to use for the daily practice sessions. Some home units can "download" onto the clinic unit; that is, they store information about practice session frequency and results, which then is transferred to the clinic computer.

Biofeedback can be used successfully if an individual is able to process information through sight or sound and make modifications based on that input. The individual needs to be motivated to learn the exercise prescribed. There are no side effects and biofeedback is non-invasive.

Biofeedback in conjunction with therapeutic exercise has been shown to be more effective and faster in diminishing incontinence than exercise alone. Biofeedback gives more accurate and fast information to the brain which improves the learning curve, increases muscle strength more quickly, and reintegrates reflex arcs more completely.

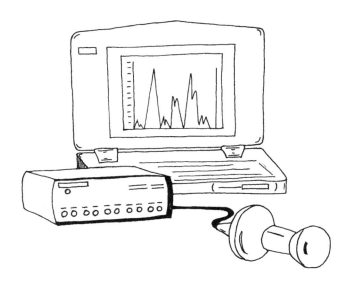

CHAPTER 13

What are Special Considerations for Special Populations?

Vulvodynia	Pregnancy
Interstitial Cystitis	Menopause
Fibromyalgia	Childhood Bedwetting
Multiple Sclerosis	Benign Prostate Hyperplasia
Diabetes	Radical Prostatectomy
	Prostatitis

Vulvodynia

Vulvodynia symptoms include complaints of burning, stinging, and irritation of the vulva and labia of the female genitalia. Even light touch or pressure around the vaginal area causes severe pain which can make it difficult to wear any clothing, to sit in any position, to ride a bicycle, to walk, or have intercourse. Urinating can cause extreme pain.

Treatment has included a low-oxalate diet, calcium citrate, an oxalate absorber, and glucosamine supplements.

Pelvic muscle exercises and biofeedback have been used successfully in cases of vulvodynia to improve pelvic muscle function and decrease pain. Physiological Quieting® is an important component to balance the autonomic nervous system and decrease pelvic muscle resting tone. Pacing daily activities, alternating rest and work cycles, and changing nutritional habits are also important.

Interstitial Cystitis

Interstitial cystitis (IC) is a chronic condition of the bladder with symptoms of severe frequency and urgency to urinate, suprapubic pressure, and pain. Toileting often occurs every 20-30 minutes during the day, instead of the normal frequency every 3 to 4 hours. Nocturia (frequent toileting at night) occurs as part of the syndrome. This can be as often as every hour and as infrequent as one to two times a night. Lower abdominal or suprapubic sensation can vary from infrequent discomfort to extreme pain which can also be in the low back, vaginal, and inner thigh regions. Sleep is significantly disrupted since toileting is so frequent, and therefore fatigue is a significant side effect. Leaking often occurs in conjunction with the urgency and frequency symptoms. Exacerbations may occur with intercourse or menstrual cycle.

Diagnosis is made by excluding other disorders, and is often verified by cystoscopic findings of diffuse hemorragic (bleeding or oozing) spots on the bladder lining. Interstitial cystitis is of unknown origin and may have several causes.

Treatment has included low dose tricyclic antidepressant medications (10-75 mg). DMSO cocktail instilled in the bladder weekly for 6-20 weeks has decreased symptoms in some individuals. Hydrodistension of the bladder (stretching the bladder using an infusion of water) is done under anesthesia and has alleviated symptoms in some cases. Bladder surgery is considered in some intractable situations.

Myofascial release, cranial-sacral therapy, and trigger point massage can relieve pain and trigger point symptoms. Electrical stimulation can also help with relief of muscle trigger points and muscle hyperactivity.

Roll for Control® exercises without resistance have been helpful in relieving symptoms of interstitial cystitis. Contracting and relaxing the pelvic muscles increases circulation to nerves and muscles of the region and can help normalize the numerous reflex arcs that coordinate the bladder and bowel system. Pelvic muscle exercise improves muscle tone and muscle function.

Physiological Quieting® with biofeedback has helped to relieve symptoms by quieting or inhibiting excessive bladder contractions and helping the pelvic muscles to relax in the resting state.

Dietary changes have also helped some individuals with IC. Avoiding acidic and spicy food and drink has alleviated some symptoms. Eliminating caffeine and consuming 6-8 glasses of fluid a day have been important dietary changes. Any constipation or other bowel problems need to be addressed through dietary changes and exercise because the bowel is integrally connected to the bladder, and any distension or irritation of the bowel causes irritation of the bladder.

Electrical stimulation intravaginally has also assisted in quieting or inhibiting the overactive bladder muscle. Individuals report decreased suprapubic and back pain as well as less frequent toileting episodes.

Fibromyalgia

Fibromyalgia is described as widespread pain of more than three months duration in combination with tender points at specific sites throughout the body. Tenderness can vary from a grimace or flinch to intolerable pain from light touch. Specific complaints often include urinary frequency, lower abdominal pain and pressure, leaking, enuresis, and interstitial cystitis-like symptoms.

Roll for Control® exercises, Physiological Quieting® and biofeedback are important components of treatment for fibromyalgia and incontinence. Medication, often tricyclic antidepressants, can be a beneficial component of treatment to gain long-term suppression of leaking.

Multiple Sclerosis

Multiple sclerosis (MS) is a neurological disorder affecting sensation, body movement, and function. Plaque formation on nerves throughout the brain and peripheral nervous system acts as a block to normal nerve transmission. The plaque may change in location and severity with time so symptoms change too. Plaque on nerves affecting the bowel and bladder are relatively common in MS. Ten percent of the time bladder symptoms are the initial symptoms leading to the MS diagnosis. Common symptoms often include urinary urgency and frequency; difficulty initiating urination; small, weak stream flow; lack of complete bladder emptying; nighttime leaking; and inability to know when to toilet.

If the plaque is affecting nerves that innervate the pelvic muscles, the symptoms include leaking of urine because the muscles are too weak or slow in reacting to hold urine in, or difficulty releasing the muscles to let all the urine flow out. Joan described that, despite her urge to go to the toilet, she had to concentrate on relaxing the pelvic muscles as she sat on the toilet so she could initiate a good stream of urine.

If the plaque is affecting the nerves that innervate the bladder and urethra, the bladder may be floppy and unable to contract enough to push the urine out, and/ or the internal sphincter may tighten excessively so the urine cannot flow down the urethra. This is called bladder-sphincter dysenergia. The result is retention of urine in the bladder and overflow incontinence or leaking at unpredictable times.

Medication, is often one of the first recommendations for treatment. It has the effect of increasing action of the bladder muscle and relaxing the internal sphincter muscle.

Physiological Quieting® with diaphragmatic breathing can assist in relaxing the pelvic muscles and normalizing autonomic nervous system messages to the bladder and urethra.

Roll for Control® exercises can be an important treatment as long as there is an understanding that the rest phase of exercise is as important as the contract phase. Exercise improves circulation and stimulates nerve muscle connections. Because fatigue is a factor in MS, short periods of exercise (3-5 minutes) are recommended.

Diabetes

Diabetes is a metabolic condition characterized by the body's inability to adequately produce and/or effectively utilize insulin. This effects every body organ in some way. The urinary consequences can include frequency and urgency of urination when blood sugars are elevated. Peripheral neuropathy can result in an atonic, floppy bladder that is unable to empty completely. Sensation can also be affected, so messages about the need to urinate are not always accurately communicated to the brain. Pelvic muscle weakness due to neuropathy and inadequate circulation can lead to leaking during daily physical activities. Excessive sugar in the urine causes bladder irritation resulting in frequent urge sensations when there is not a full bladder.

The most important treatment for bladder symptoms in diabetes is maintenance of good control of blood sugar levels through medication, regular exercise, a balanced diet, and regular blood glucose monitoring.

The Roll for Control® exercises can be very beneficial to re-educate the pelvic and urogential diaphragm muscles and normalize the bladder muscle's function. A maintenance level of exercise is usually 5-10 minutes daily.

Physiological Quieting® is beneficial in blood glucose regulation and in bladder function, so a 20 minute session once a day is recommended.

Pregnancy

The anatomical and physiological changes during pregnancy predispose the woman to incontinence episodes. As pregnancy progresses, the uterus enlarges to accommodate the growing fetus and this puts pressure on the bladder. The ligamentous and fascial supportive structures relax during pregnancy to allow the uterus to grow and to enable the pelvis to expand for a vaginal delivery. Secondarily, the ligaments and fascia cannot support the bladder and bladder angle as effectively. Constipation is often a problem in the last trimester (3 months) of pregnancy due to the crowded conditions in the pelvis and the physiological change in contractility of the lower bowel. Constipation causes increased irritation of the bladder which can precipitate leaking.

During childbirth, the pudendal nerve, that innervates the pelvic muscles, can be traumatized so there is dysfunction of the muscle-nerve connection. The pelvic muscles are stretched and sometimes injured during the delivery process. Relaxation of the ligamentous and fascial structures continues for several months after the delivery or until breastfeeding ceases. The structures of the lower pelvis, bladder, uterus, and bowel have been pushed lower in the pelvis during delivery. Postpartum, approximately 20% of women experience leaking.

Physiological Quieting® is beneficial during pregnancy, labor and postpartum. Roll for Control® exercises help prepare the pelvic muscles for delivery and are important to use postpartum for recovery of muscle tone and function. Lifestyle Changes including sleep, nutrition and walking will assist the individual in maintaining optimal health for the baby and the mother. Inversion on the Wonder W'edge™ is often helpful to realign internal organs and muscles, especially if the woman is experiencing back pain or constipation. (Fig. 13-1) Always check with your physician before doing any new exercise.

During the delivery process, the woman assists by bearing down or pushing to help the fetus descend into the birth canal. The most efficient method to accomplish this involves a coordination of voluntary activity between the abdominal, breathing diaphragm, and pelvic muscles. The breathing diaphragm is set in a lowered position while the abdominal muscles tighten to increase intra-abdominal pressure and the pelvic muscles are relaxed so the baby can be pushed out.

Menopause

When a woman ceases menstruating, physical changes associated with hormonal changes occur. The pelvic muscles, connective tissue, fascia, and ligaments are estrogen dependent. As estrogen decreases with menopause, the pelvic tissues become dry, thin, and less elastic. The bladder and bowel and pelvic muscles descend lower in the pelvis as the supportive structures relax and thin. The bladder becomes more irritable. The result can be urge and/or stress incontinence. The bowel becomes more sluggish. The result can be constipation.

Bladder and bowel problems in this age group are most often treated conservatively with exercise and medication after a medical evaluation. The Roll for Control® exercises performed 3-5 minutes daily is recommended as a preventive exercise program for women after the age of 40 to maintain pelvic muscle strength and bladder support. Using the Wonder W'edge™ to elevate the hips during roll in and out exercises is beneficial for optimal position of the bladder and uterus. (Fig. 13-1) Physiological Quieting®, for short periods throughout the day helps normalize bladder and bowel muscle activity so urge sensations are decreased. Walking 30 minutes daily helps maintain bone strength, heart, lung and bladder health.

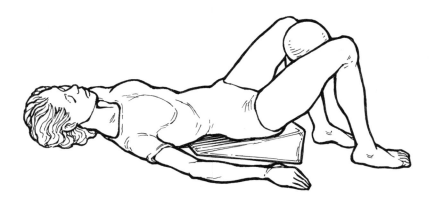

Figure 13-1

Childhood Nighttime Wetting - Nocturnal Enuresis

Children are usually dry at night between the ages of 3 and 4. After 8 years old, frequent leaking is considered abnormal, but in reality it is relatively common; approximately 5 percent of 10 year olds and 1 to 2 percent of adults still leak at night. Twice as many boys than girls experience the problem. Nocturnal enuresis tends to run in families. It is unusual for nighttime wetting in children to be due to medical problems, but there should be a check for urinary tract infection, diabetes, or an anatomic abnormality. Nighttime wetting can also result from emotional trauma, such as separation from a parent or abuse, but most of the time it is not a psychologically caused problem. Some children have a small bladder capacity and may be helped by increased fluid intake and bladder training (to wait before urinating for increasing periods of time).

In general, nocturnal enuresis in children can be regarded as the need to learn a developmental skill that did not come automatically for these children, and for the pelvic muscles and bladder muscle to mature in tone and coordination in order to function at a more sophisticated level at night as well as during the day.

Bed wetting will often cause increased tension in the family. Someone or something is sometimes blamed for the behavior. The child, as well as the rest of the family, needs to understand that bed wetting is not usually intentional; and is not a result of laziness or not caring. In most cases, if parents are calm and patient, the problem can be effectively treated.

Treatment includes the Beyond Kegel® Protocol:
1) Lifestyle Changes
2) Physiological Quieting® for Kids
3) Roll for Control® Exercises

Lifestyle Changes

Lifestyle Changes include fluid intake, a constipation reducing program, and behavioral techniques to train awakening to toilet. One of the first things parents and children commonly do to "cure" nighttime wetting is to decrease the amount of fluid the child is consuming. The result is that the bladder (detrusor) muscle "shrinks" and can hold less and less before it lets the brain know it is time to urinate. This decrease in fluid intake also causes more concentrated waste products in the urine which is irritating to the bladder lining. Decreased fluid intake can cause dehydration which affects all body functions. Instead of limiting fluids, the child should drink 4-6 eight-ounce glasses of appropriate fluid a day. Appropriate fluids include water, fruit juice, and milk. Caffeine is irritating to the bladder and the nervous system, so colas, coffee, and tea are not recommended. If the child drinks eight ounces of fluid with each meal, and a small bike bottle of fluid between meals, the amount is adequate. Stop drinking after dinner.

A nutrition program to prevent constipation is another important lifestyle change to consider. A significant number of children bedwet secondary to constipation. A nutrition program for an improved bowel pattern can be as simple as adding a fresh pear or peach a day and fresh spinach with extra virgin olive oil to the meals. Other times a normal bowel pattern is obtained by eliminating white bread, rice and pasta.

Behavioral techniques to train awakening at night to toilet is another lifestyle change. Parents often try to cure bed wetting by carrying the sleeping child to the toilet when the parents go to bed. This may prevent wetting, but it does not help the child to have independent control. It is essential that the child awaken and make the connection between waking and the desire to urinate. An enuresis alarm and a star chart enables the child to learn this skill in a positive way.

Physiological Quieting® for Kids

Balancing the autonomic nervous system is important in nighttime bed wetting for several reasons. It can facilitate normalizing day and nighttime bladder and bowel patterns. It can improve sleep patterns. It can balance emotional variations when dealing with bladder problems.

PQ for Kids is a CD with five short activities that help children balance their autonomic nervous system. The activities are fun and easy to do. Special needs children including those with autism, Aspergers and attention deficit hyperactivity disorder have benefited from use of this CD.

Roll for Control® Exercises

Roll for Control® exercises improve the coordination of the pelvic muscles with the bladder and bowel system. Assisted Pelvic Muscle Tightening- Roll In and Out and Standing Plié exercises can be done twice daily for 5-10 repetitions each time.

The Beyond Kegels® Protocol usually takes between 2-6 weeks to achieve continence at night. Enuresis may reoccur months or years after the "cure," when the child has undergone a growth spurt or has had the flu or other systemic illness. If this happens, a "refresher course" of 1-2 weeks is usually adequate for a return to normal. The book, "Bladder and Bowel Issues for Kids", provides more detailed information.

Male
Benign Prostate Hyperplasia
Radical Prostatectomy
Prostatitis

Urinary incontinence in men is usually experienced after age 60 and often is related to prostate enlargement, whether benign or cancerous.

Benign Prostate Hyperplasia

Prostate enlargement can be benign/nonmalignant and this is termed benign prostate hyperplasia. As the prostate enlarges, it can occlude or narrow the urethra so urine cannot flow out effectively and efficiently, even though the bladder may be contracting to push the urine out and the internal and external sphincter muscles are relaxed to release urine. When this obstruction occurs, the symptoms can include a weak stream of urine, frequent feelings of urge to urinate but only small amounts of urine are released, relatively small leaks of urine during physical activity, and/or occasional large leaking episodes when there is the urge to toilet and it has been several hours since the last toileting and/or a considerable fluid intake.

Urethral blockage by the prostate can cause incomplete emptying of the bladder. The medical term for this is post void residual (PVR). This can lead to a bladder infection, irritated bladder lining, or urine reflux into the kidneys.

Radical Prostatectomy

In cancerous enlargement of the prostate gland, radical prostatectomy is often recommended. This is complete removal of the prostate gland and related tissue in the hope of eliminating all cancerous cells. In some cases, pelvic lymph nodes are also removed. Other treatment options include radiation and hormonal therapy including removal of the testicles to eliminate testosterone. A result of these treatment approaches can be total or partial urinary incontinence.

Chronic Prostatitis

Chronic benign prostatitis causes pain in the male genitalia and pelvic region. It can also lead to urgency and frequency, discomfort during urination and poor urine flow.

The Beyond Kegels® Protocol is beneficial for men with benign prostate hyperplasia, radical prostatectomy or chronic prostatitis. Treatment includes:
1) Lifestyle Changes
2) Physiological Quieting®
3) Roll for Control® Exercises
4) Wonder W'edge Inversion

Lifestyle changes

Lifestyle changes include fluid intake, walking, and nutrition to normalize bowel patterns.

Fluids: One of the first actions often taken by men experiencing urinary incontinence is to decrease fluid intake throughout the day and night. The immediate result of this may be a little less leaking but the long term result can be devastating. Less fluid in the bladder causes the bladder to shrink because it responds to the volume of liquid by adjusting in size much like a balloon enlarges as it is filled with air. A smaller bladder means it sends more frequent messages to the brain that it needs to empty. Eventually the individual can be toileting every 30 minutes during the day and hourly at night.

Less urine means the urine is more concentrated and often more irritating to the bladder lining. This can cause the bladder to contract more frequently and strongly, so some men describe experiencing an explosion of urine they cannot control. Concentrated urine can lead to bladder and lower abdominal discomfort and even bladder infections.

It is important that 6-8 glasses of non-caffeinated fluid be consumed daily. It is appropriate to stop fluids after 6:00 p.m. to facilitate longer periods between toileting during the night. The fluid intake is best if it is spread out evenly through the day.

Walking: Walking 30-40 minutes a day is essential to return the pelvic muscles and bladder and bowel to normal function. Men often stop walking when leaking increases with physical activity. It is important to use appropriate protective pads and continue walking and participating in other physical and recreational activities.

Men comment that they do not go out socially or they curtail physical activity because they fear leaking will be obvious due to staining or odor. Appropriate pads can alleviate these fears. Adhesive backed pads attach to underwear. Disposable undergarments are available through the mail or in grocery stores or pharmacies.

Nutrition: Constipation is common with prostate growth, surgery and pain. A nutrition program for an improved bowel pattern can be as simple as adding a fresh pear or peach a day and fresh spinach with extra virgin olive oil to the meals. Other times a normal bowel pattern is obtained by reducing white bread, rice and pasta.

Physiological Quieting®

Men unconsciously tighten the pelvic muscles when there is pain or dysfunction in the urinary or bowel systems. The increased tone can lead to increased symptoms and a continued downhill spiral. Sleep is disrupted, social and job relationships are impacted.

Equal to exercise as a priority, Physiological Quieting®, can normalize pelvic muscle tone and assist the return of bladder and bowel function. Use the Physiological Quieting® CD at night and practice diaphragmatic breathing and handwarming hourly for 30 seconds.

Roll for Control® Exercises

The exercises described in this book are appropriate for men. Begin with 3-5 repetitions and progress to 10 repetitions 3 times a day. More is not better.

Treatment duration for men who have had radical prostatectomies and radiation may be longer than the typical incontinence treatment program of 4-8 weeks of exercise. Improvement has been noted over a 12-month exercise program, possibly due to nerve and muscle regeneration and healing. Once the exercise progression is completed (usually in 4-6 weeks), the individual is seen once every 4-8 weeks for follow- up and alterations to the program. An important aspect of the follow-up visits with these individuals is encouragement to continue the regular exercise protocol, fluid intake, and lifestyle changes.

Men will ask if the exercises can improve impotence if that has been a result of surgery or radiation. There are no objective findings to indicate that exercise can reverse this problem, but the stimulation to all body systems, including circulatory, hormonal, and neurological, can only be positive for the body healing itself.

CHAPTER 14

What Medications Can Help?

Medications have been shown to be beneficial in treating urinary incontinence. In conjunction with exercise and behavioral strategies, they are recommended as the first step in treating incontinence in the Clinical Practice Guideline published by the Department of Health and Human Services, 1996.

Short term medication trials benefit some patients with urge incontinence, but the side effects can be significant and research indicates that few individuals become symptom-free.

Medication use may improve symptoms in approximately half of the individuals with stress or mixed incontinence, but again few become symptom-free. Medications used for stress incontinence have fewer side effects than those used for urge incontinence.

Medications used for overflow incontinence exhibit significant side effects, and improvement in symptoms varies.

Medication use should be based on individual patient needs, ie., contraindications, cost, and drug interactions. Initial dosages in most medications used for incontinence should be low and increased slowly.

Pharmacologic treatment for urinary incontinence is an important component of treatment but needs to be used in combination with exercise, behavioral and sometimes surgical strategies.

Description of Commonly Used Medications
Urge Incontinence
Anticholinergic Agents

Function: Decreases bladder contractions, relaxes smooth muscle

Effect: Decreases urge incontinence leaking, increases bladder capacity, increases time between voiding

Examples	*Dose*
oxybutynin (Ditropan XL)	2.5-5 mg 1-4x/day
propantheline (Pro-Banthine)	7.5-30 mg, 15-60mg
dicyclomine hydrochloride (Bentyl)	20 mg 4x/day
hyoscyamine (Levsin)	0.125-0.25 mg
tolterodine tartrate(Detrol LA)	2-4 mg 1x/day

Side effects: Dry skin, blurred vision, change in mental state, drowsiness, confusion, nausea, constipation, dry mouth, tachycardia (increased heart rate), weakness, orthostatic hypotension (low blood pressure on arising from reclining)

Note: Should not be used if narrow angle glaucoma is present.

Estrogen Replacement Therapy (ERT)

Function: Restore urethral mucosa, increase vascularity, tone and responsiveness of urethral muscle, increase alpha adrenergic receptors of urethra

Effect: Improve internal sphincter function, decrease incontinence with increased intra-abdominal pressure, decreases irritative voiding symptoms, decreases frequency of urination especially at night

Examples	Dose
conjugated estrogen (Premarin)	0.623-1. 25 mg daily

Side Effects: Not recommended for women with a history of breast or uterine cancer, blood clots, or liver damage

Tricyclic Antidepressant Agents (TCA)

Function: Increases CNS serotonin neurotransmitter levels

Effect: Reduces daytime leaking, reduces nighttime leaking

Examples	Dose
imipramine (Tofranil)	10-25 mg 1-4x/day
doxepin (Sinequan)	10-50 mg 3x/day
desipramine (Norpramin)	25 mg 1-3x/day
nortriptyline (Pamelor)	10-25 mg 1-3x/day
amitriptyline (Elavil)	10-25 mg 3-4x/day

Side effects: cardiac alterations, anticholinergic effects, fatigue, xerostomia, dizziness, blurred vision

Stress Incontinence

Alpha Adrenergic Agonists

Function: Affects receptors at bladder neck, internal sphincter, and proximal urethra causing increased muscle tone in this area

Effect: Decreases leaking with intra-abdominal pressure, tightens bladder outlet muscle

Examples	Dose
phenylpropanolamine (PPA) (Dexatrim)	25-50 mg 4x/day
psuedoephedrine (Sudafed)	30-60 mg 4x/day

Side Effects: Nausea, xerostomia, insomnia, restlessness, anxiety, headache, hypertension, heart palpitations

Note: Not to be used in people with increased blood pressure/hypertension, severe congestive heart failure, cardiac arrhythmias

Estrogen Replacement Therapy(ERT)

Function: Restore urethral mucosa, increase vascularity, tone and responsiveness of urethral muscle, increase alpha adrenergic receptors of urethra

Effect: Improve internal sphincter function, decrease incontinence with increased intra-abdominal pressure, decreases irritative voiding symptoms, decreases frequency of urination especially at night

Examples	Dose
conjugated estrogen (Premarin)	0.623-1. 25 mg daily

Side Effects: Not recommended for women with a history of breast or uterine cancer, blood clots, or liver damage

Combination Therapy- ERT and PPA

Recommended in stress incontinence in post-menopausal women if single drug therapy has proven inadequate

Tricyclic Antidepressant Agents

Example	Dose
imipramine (Tofranil)	5-75 mg/day

(See description under Urge Incontinence medications.)

(Propranolol and other beta blockers are not recommended at this time due to lack of clinical research.)

Antidiurectic Hormone

Example	Dose
desmopressin (DDAVP)	

Effect: Decreases nocturnal enuresis (nighttime wetting) and nighttime polyuria; at this time used for children only

Overflow Incontinence

Alpha Adrenergic Antagonists

Function: Relaxes internal sphincter muscle

Effect: Increases outlet size causing improved flow of urine, decreased residual urine, decreased leaking due to more complete emptying

Examples	Dose
terazosin (Hytrin)	1 mg daily
prazosin (Minipress)	1 mg 2-3x/daily
doxazosin (Cardura)	1 mg daily

Side Effects: Orthostatic hypotension (which can lead to falls, should be taken at bedtime), tachycardia (increased heart rate)

Cholinergic Agonists

Function: Increases bladder muscle contractions

Effect: Increases force with which bladder muscle pushes urine down and out the urethra, decreases residual urine, decreases leaking because of more complete emptying

Example	Dose
bethanechol (Urecholine)	10-50 mg 2-4x/day

Side Effects: flushing, abdominal cramps, diarrhea, nausea and vomiting, sweating, salivation

Medications that Cause Incontinence Symptoms

Many of the same medications used to treat incontinence can also cause incontinence if used inappropriately. Medications used to treat other conditions can have side effects that cause incontinence.

Medication	Possible Side Effects
Sedatives/Hypnotics	sedation, immobility, muscle relaxation,
CNS Depressants diazepan (Valium) flurazepam (Dalmane) alcohol	delirium, frequency and urgency leaking
Diuretics furosemide (Lasix) bumetanide (Bumex) loop diuretics	polyuria, frequency and urgency leaking
Antipsychotics thioridazine (Mellaril) haloperidol (Haldol)	sedation, rigidity, immobility, urge and overflow leaking, anticholinergic actions
Antidepressants imiprimine (Tofranil) doxepin (Sinequan) desipramine (Norpramin) amitriptyline (Elavil)	fatique, dizziness, bladder relaxation, constipation
Anti-Parkinson Agents benztropine (Cogentin) trihexyphenidyl (Artane)	bladder relaxation, urge and overflow leaking

Medication	Possible Side Effects

Anticholinergic Agents
    antihistamines-
    diphenhydramine (Benadryl)
    hydroxyzine (Vistaril, Atarax)
	sedation, urine retention, weak stream, frequency, urge and overflow leaking, fecal impaction

Alpha Adrenergic Agonist Agents
    phenylpropranolamine
        (Ephedrine)
	sedation, urine retention, weak stream, frequency, urge and overflow leaking

Alpha Adrenergic Antagonist Agents
    prazosin (Minipress)
    terazosin (Hytrin)
    doxazosin (Cardura)
	urethral relaxation, leak with cough/ sneeze/laugh

Calcium Channel Blocking Agents
    nifedipine (Adalat, Procardia)
    diltiazem (Cardizem)
	urine retention, fluid retention, bladder (detrusor) relaxation

Narcotic Analgesic Agents morphine, etc.	urine retention, sedation, delirium constipation, impaction
Anti-hypertensive Agents	bladder and sphincter relaxation
Caffeine	aggravation or precipitation of leaking

CHAPTER 15

How Did the Beyond Kegels® Protocol Help? Case Studies Revisited

Case Studies
What Did Exercise Do To Help?

Remember the case studies at the beginning of this book in Chapter 3? Go back now, review the histories and outline the recommendations you would have for each individual to become continent and/or resume regular daily acitivities.

What Lifestyle Changes would you recommend?

What Roll for Control® exercises, Physiological Quieting® and Wonder W'edge™ Inversion will help them and why?

How often should they do the Roll for Control®, exercises, Physiological Quieting®, Wonder W'edge™ Inversion?

What is success?

Then, read this chapter to see how each individual took back the control of incontinence and returned to a fullfilling daily life.

Lizzie, 9 years old: Bed wetting

Lizzie, 9 years old, was seen for 3 visits over a 6-week period. She carried out the nocturnal enuresis exercise and alarm protocol. Within 3 weeks she was dry at night.

She has been followed for 3 years. There has been a return of symptoms once after a growth spurt. She went back on the program for 2 weeks and has been dry since then.

Mary, 29 years old: Stress Incontinence

Mary, 29 years old, was seen for 10 visits over a 4-month period of time. She practiced Physiological Quieting® morning and night. Exercises included the Roll for Control® exercises for incontinence and lumbar stabilization exercises for low back pain. Lifestyle changes were also a major emphasis in her treatment program. Initially she began a paced aerobic exercise program, 30 minutes daily followed by lumbar stabilization exercises and a rest period of 30 minutes. She changed her work schedule to two three-hour work shifts instead of 6 continuous hours of work. Between the 3 hour shifts, she did her exercise, rested, and ate lunch which she used to skip.

Three weeks after beginning the exercise and lifestyle change protocol, Mary was toileting every 3-4 hours during the day and once a night. At 4 weeks she was dry during the day except when running. Back pain significantly decreased within six weeks. She was on an independent exercise program for the last six weeks.

At discharge she was continent during all activities. She was working full-time and exercising daily without problems.

Erin, 32 years old: Stress Incontinence

Erin, 32 years old, was seen for 3 visits in 4 weeks. Her treatment protocol included the Beyond Kegels ®Protocol. She eliminated caffeine and increased her water consumption. She practice Roll for Control® exercises three times a day on the Wonder W'edge™. Erin was dry during aerobics within three weeks.

Beth, 59 years old: Urge Incontinence

Beth, 59 years old, was seen for 4 visits. She was totally continent in 3 weeks. Her treatment protocol included adequate fluid intake, no caffeine, daily aerobic exercise for 30 minutes, and the Roll for Control® exercises on the Wonder W'edge™ twice daily and Physiological Quieting® hourly.

Matilda, 82 years old: Stress Incontinence

Matilda, 82 years old, was seen for 3 visits over a 6-week period. Her treatment included the Beyond Kegels® Protocol. Lifestyle changes included adequate fluid intake, and eliminating caffeine. She changed from tea to hot lemon water. She used the Wonder W'edge™ for the Roll for Control® exercises twice a day. She practiced Physiological Quieting® at night using the CD.

At discharge she was dry at night and usually dry during the day. She wore a mini-pad during the day because she "felt safer that way." She felt confident wearing dresses and going to church or out to lunch with her family.

Robert, 75 years old: Radical Prostatectomy

Robert, 75 years old, was seen for 12 visits over a 9 month period of time. Initially his treatment protocol included Physiological Quieting® to quiet the pelvic muscles. They were in constant contraction in an attempt to stop the leaking. Lifestyle changes included adequate fluid intake and eliminating caffeine. He began taking walks again for 15 minute periods. He rested midday for 45-60 minutes.

Within 3 weeks, Robert was beginning the Roll for Control® exercises. His progress was slow but steady for the next 6 weeks. He could begin to feel the leaks, and his urine stream flow was stronger.

After 8 weeks, Robert was seen every 6-8 weeks for follow up and reinforcement to continue the exercise routine. He continued to have gradually less leaking. After 9 months he was totally dry and had resumed all activities. His only comment was that he had to get his rest or he noticed his urine control was not as good.

Barron, 86 years old: Urge Incontinence

Barron, 86 years old, was seen for 4 visits. He followed the Beyond Kegels® Protocol, increased his fluid intake to 6-8 glasses a day, and practiced spacing his toileting every 2-3 hours. He practiced Roll for Control® exercises twice a day and Physiological Quieting® hourly as often as he could remember it. He continued being physically active. Leaking decreased significantly and the explosions were eliminated. He occasionally leaked small amounts with heavy lifting or getting up after sitting in a meeting for several hours.

Ken, 55 years old: Constipation

Ken, 55 years old, was seen for 3 visits. He followed the Beyond Kegels® Protocol. Lifestyle changes included a fresh pear and spinach salad with extra virgin olive oil dressing daily. He eliminated white bread, rice and pasta. He consumed 6-8 glasses of water a day and eliminated all but two cups of coffee each day. Ken practiced Physiological Quieting® at bedtime using the CD. He practiced Roll for Control® exercises on the Wonder W'edge™ every morning and evening. Ken began walking in the evening for 20-30 minutes. Within three weeks he was having soft, formed stools eliminated without straining on an every day basis. He described feeling no abdominal discomfort and a higher energy level. His hemorrhoids were gone and the urinary urgency was rare.

Lillie, 24 years old: Diarrhea

Lillie, 24 years old, was seen for 6 visits. She followed the Beyond Kegels® Protocol although it was hard to be consistent with her busy schedule. She reported doing well with the program 3-4 days a week. Lifestyle changes included changing her diet to foods that move more slowly through the intestines. She changed breakfast to cooked oatmeal with apple and banana 3 days a week. She added white rice, potato or pasta to lunch or dinner. She continued the same drinking schedule. Lillie practiced Physiological Quieting® between her aerobics classes for 3-4 minutes 3 times a day. She practiced the Roll for Control® exercises as part of the classes she taught at the health club. Lillie noticed improvement within 2 weeks but then fell off her program and the diarrhea came back. She "got serious" about changing for her lifetime and by 4 weeks she was experiencing diarrhea once a week. By the 5th week she went a week with normal bowel movements.

In Summary

There are common threads in the programs of all the individuals who shared their stories even though each problem was unique.

All individuals understood the basic concepts of anatomy and function of the bladder and bowel systems. They understood the neurological connection between the brain, spinal cord and bladder and bowel systems. They understood the possibilities for voluntary control of both systems.

All individuals used self care strategies during daily activities. They became more attentive to their physical needs. Sometimes it was less caffeine and more clear liquid. Other times it was rest in the middle of the day.

All individuals were reliable in carrying out an exercise program on a daily basis. The exercise program re-educated the pelvic muscles to efficiently rest or relax as well as act appropriately during daily activities. The exercise program strengthened the pelvic muscles so they could support the bladder and bowel in optimum positions for continence. Many individuals use the Wonder W'edge Inversion™ to re-aligh internal organs and the spine.

Most individuals utilized Physiological Quieting® to normalize the tone and function of the bladder (detrusor muscle) and bowel and to improve the resting level of pelvic muscles which is as important as the ability to contract or tighten them.

These therapeutic approaches are as beneficial for individuals before they experience a problem as a preventive protocol as for the individuals with incontinence problems. Many clients say, "I told my friend to start doing the Fabulous Four Exercises and get rid of coffee now so she won't ever have the problem I have. It's just good sense for long life!"

The next chapter will help you carry out your customized program.

May you have a long, happy, and active life.

CHAPTER 16

Set Your Goals and Practice Your Program

What do you want to accomplish while doing the Beyond Kegels® Bladder and Bowel Health Program? First answer the questions in the Bladder and Bowel Health Questionnaire from Chapter 2. Next, go to page 154 and evaluate the results from this baseline data. Now it's time to set the goals you want to achieve. If you are drinking caffeine set your goal to decrease the amount of caffeine 1-2 cups per day. If you are not drinking enough fluid each day set your goal for 1-2 more glasses of fluid each day in a 1-2 week period. If you have frequency increase, count the number of toiletings a day and set your goal for 1-2 fewer toiletings per day in a 1-2 week period. If you have stress incontinence problems count the number of leaks per day and the number of pads you are using, then set your goal for 1-2 fewer leaks in 1-2 weeks and 1 less pad per day in 1-2 weeks. If you have urge incontinence problems count the number of urges and the number of leaks, then set your goal for 1-2 fewer urges and leaks per day in 1-2 weeks time. If you have stopped some daily recreational, work or home activities, set your goal to start the activity again for a short period, taking small steps toward your larger goal.

You may do somewhat better or worse than each goal because everyone is different but this gives you a place to start and lets you know how you are progressing. Now that you have set your goals you can begin your personal plan of action.

You will do the Lifestyle Changes, Physiological Quieting® and Roll for Control® exercises every day to obtain the quickest improvement in the least amount of time. It is important that you do not overdo the exercises since you are doing them every day. More is not better in this case, so do just the number of repetitions suggested. Record your exercise sessions on the daily activity record.

Every week take a day to record on the bladder/bowel diary. Then enter that information on the Comparison Data Record. Note any changes that have occurred since you last recorded information. Evaluate your progress and make a decision about next week's program. For example if you are making progress continue with the same program and add the new week's suggestions when you feel comfortable that the previous activities are easy to do. If your are not making progress or the exercises are difficult then remain at the same activity level and look at the other activities that can be just as important in helping to achieve your goals. For instance coffee consumption and Physiological Quieting® are activities that can significantly affect your bladder and bowel health.

Continue with the weekly programs until you are symptom free, the problems you check off in the questionnaire are resolved and you have accomplished your goals as completely as possible. When you have achieved a normal bladder and bowel health pattern for 2 weeks proceed to the Maintenance Program.

Baseline Data

The first few days you will keep track of your behavior including toileting, drinking fluids, consuming caffeine, any leaking incidences, and use of protective pads. This baseline data will tell you if the Beyond Kegels® Protocol is helping. You will compare each week's data while you are carrying out the bladder and bowel health program with the baseline data. So we recommend keeping three days of baseline data before starting the Beyond Kegels® program. If that seems impossible try doing just one day or two half days, one half day in the morning and one half day in the afternoon/evening.

1. Next, record the baseline data on the following page. Put a T whenever you use the toilet to urinate. Record a B when you have a bowel movement, a BC for constipation, a BD for diarrhea. Record an F when you drink 8 ounces of fluid Mark the F with a * when the fluid is caffeinated. Record an L if you leak a little and an A if you experience a large leak. Record a P when you use a new protective pad. Then summarize the data on the Comparison Sheet on page 168.

2. Evaluate bladder and bowel baseline data and the Bladder and Bowel Health Questionnaire results. The baseline data and questionnaire data are very important. They help you analyze where to start and let you set goals for where you want to be. Compare your information with the Normal Bladder and Bowel Health Patterns. Then set your goals.

My Goals:

1. _____

2. _____

3. _____

4. _____

Now you are ready to start your program.

BASELINE
Bladder/Bowel Diary

Name

Day _____ *Date* _____		*Day* _____ *Date* _____	
6-8am	_____	*6-8am*	_____
8-10	_____	*8-10*	_____
10-12	_____	*10-12*	_____
12-2pm	_____	*12-2pm*	_____
2-4	_____	*2-4*	_____
4-6	_____	*4-6*	_____
6-8	_____	*6-8*	_____
8-10	_____	*8-10*	_____
10-12	_____	*10-12*	_____
overnight	_____	*overnight*	_____
*pads used	_____	**pads used*	_____
comments	_____	*comments*	_____

T=toilet   *F-8oz. fluid*
L=small leak   **=caffeinated*
A=large leak   *P=pad*
B=bowel movement
BC=bowel movement constipation
BD= bowel movement diarrhea

155

Beyond Kegels Program- Week One

During this first week you will make Lifestyle Changes, begin Physiological Quieting® and Roll for Control® exercises.

☐ **1. Lifestyle Change - Sleep and Nutrition**

☐ A. Sleep 8-9 hours/night on a regular schedule.

☐ B. Drink 6-8 eight ounce glasses of non-caffeinated fluid each day. Spread the fluid intake throughout the day.

☐ C. Eliminate caffeine: coffee, tea, colas, and chocolate.

Eliminate caffeine gradually. If you drink coffee or colas you might want to change to decaffeinated and gradually decrease the caffeine that way. Then decrease the decaffeinated coffee or cola gradually since it has chemicals that can be somewhat irritating to the bladder and influence frequency. If you consume many cups of caffeine you may need to take 2 weeks to change to non-caffeinated beverages since rebound headaches can occur with faster removal of caffeine.

☐ D. Change food choices depending on bowel movement patterns. If you experience a constipation pattern add fresh fruit like a pear, peach or plums, and vegetables like fresh spinach, broccoli, or chard. If you experience a diarrhea pattern add fresh fruit like a banana or apple and white rice, pasta and bread.

☐ 2. Physiological Quieting®

☐ A. Diaphramatic Breathing - practice 3-4 times per day for 6-7 breaths.

☐ B. Handwarming - Practice 3-4 times per day for 30-60 seconds.

☐ 3. Roll For Control® Exercises

This first week you will also begin the Roll for Control® Exercises to improve muscle control of bladder and bowel function. Repeat the following sequence 2-3 times a day. Pick times during the day that are good for you and when you won't feel hurried.

☐ Roll for Control® Exercise #1
Relaxed Awareness

Relax into the support of the chair or bed. Release all your muscles from head to toes into the support. Notice your slow, low breathing -- inhale then exhale -- and maintain this breathing rhythm throughout all the exercises. Focus on this exercise for 30-60 seconds.

☐ Roll for Control® Exercise #2-O
Roll Out – Obturator Assist

Roll out against Roll for Control® band.

A. Secure the Roll for Control band® around your legs just above the knees while you squeeze your thighs together. Fasten the band with the Roll for Control clippie. Position your heels touching each other.

B. Focus on your slow low breathing and maintain that breathing throughout the exercise.

C. Separate you knees 3-4 inches, rolling them out against the band. At the same time, rotate your toes apart like a windshield wiper, while keeping your heels touching.

D. Hold your knees apart, pushing against the band for a slow count of 10.

E. Return to the knees together and feet together position and rest for a slow count of 10.

F. Repeat this exercise for 10 repetitions 2-3 times daily.

4. Wonder W'edge™ Inversion

☐ Position on the Wonder W'edge 1-2 times a day for 3-5 minutes.

☐ Practice diaphragmatic breathing and Roll for Control® excercises on wedge.

5. Record Keeping.

☐ On the Daily Activity record, indicate when you perform the Roll for Control® exercises, Physiological Quieting® and when you drink fluids. Pick one day to record data on the Progress Report just like you kept during your baseline data recording. Write any comments you have in the comment section.

WEEKLY PROGRESS REPORT - WEEK ONE

Daily Activity Record Insert a slash (/) for every exercise session, P for Physiological Quieting and an F for every glass of fluid you drink.

MON	TUE	WED	THUR	FRI	SAT	SUN

Bladder/Bowel Diary

Name

Day_____ Date_____

6-8am	_____
8-10	_____
10-12	_____
12-2pm	_____
2-4	_____
4-6	_____
6-8	_____
8-10	_____
10-12	_____
overnight	_____
*pads used	_____
comments	_____

Day_____ Date_____

6-8am	_____
8-10	_____
10-12	_____
12-2pm	_____
2-4	_____
4-6	_____
6-8	_____
8-10	_____
10-12	_____
overnight	_____
*pads used	_____
comments	_____

T=toilet
L=small leak
A=large leak
B=bowel movement
BC=bowel movement constipation
BD= bowel movement diarrhea

F-8oz. fluid
*=caffeinated
P=pad

BEYOND KEGELS PROGRAM – WEEK TWO

During week two you will add the following activities to those you have been doing.

☐ 1. **Lifestyle Change - Nutrition and Walking**
  ☐ Add fruits and vegetables to improve bowel patterns.
  ☐ Walk 30 minutes a day.

☐ 2. **Roll for Control® Exercise #2-A**
  (Roll in Adductor Assist)
  A. Place the Roll for Control® ball between your legs just above the knees.
  B. Focus on your slow low breathing and maintain that breathing throughout the exercise.
  C. Bring your knees together, rolling them in against the Roll for Control® ball. At the same time, rotate your toes together like a windshield wiper with your heels hip-width apart.
  D. Hold your knees together, pushing against the ball for a slow count of 10.
  E. Return to the knees-apart position and rest for a slow count of 10.
  F. Repeat this exercise for 10 repetitions 2-3 times daily.

☐ 3. Physiological Quieting®

Listen to the Physiological Quieting CD at least once a day. If you are busy during the day you can listen to it at night as you go to sleep. Even if you fall asleep before it is over you still learn through the first few levels of sleep. Learning while you sleep is OK.

☐ 4. Positive Self Statements (PSST)

PSSTs are thoughts that direct chemical and electrical messages to help the bladder function normally. You can make up your own PSSTs. Here are some examples:

"I deserve to be healthy and dry. I am health and dry." "I deserve to be active and dry. I am active and dry." "I deserve to sleep through the night and be dry. I sleep through the night and am dry." Repeat PSSTs frequently through out the day, for example 10 times when you awaken, when you go to bed, while you are driving, or before eating.

My PSSTs:

1._____

2._____

3._____

WEEKLY PROGRESS REPORT - WEEK TWO

Daily Activity Record Insert a slash (/) for every exercise session, P for Physiological Quieting and an F for every glass of fluid you drink.

MON	TUE	WED	THUR	FRI	SAT	SUN

Bladder/Bowel Diary

Name _____

Day_____ Date_____	Day_____ Date_____
6-8am _____	6-8am _____
8-10 _____	8-10 _____
10-12 _____	10-12 _____
12-2pm _____	12-2pm _____
2-4 _____	2-4 _____
4-6 _____	4-6 _____
6-8 _____	6-8 _____
8-10 _____	8-10 _____
10-12 _____	10-12 _____
overnight _____	overnight _____
*pads used _____	*pads used _____
comments _____	comments _____

T=toilet
L=small leak
A=large leak
B=bowel movement
BC=bowel movement constipation
BD= bowel movement diarrhea

F-8oz. fluid
*=caffeinated
P=pad

BEYOND KEGELS PROGRAM – WEEK THREE

During week three you will add the following activities to those you have previously been doing.

1. Lifestyle Change - Social, Work, Recreation

☐ Evaluate your social and recreational activities and increase their frequency as your confidence improves.

Social and recreational activities I like to do:

1._____

2._____

3._____

4._____

2. Physiological Quieting®

☐ Practice diaphragmatic breathing and handwarming together hourly. Think "Slow, low breathing, my hands are warmer and warmer." repeat 5-6 times.

3. Roll for Control® Exercise #3
(Heel Clicks)

A. Sit with your feet hip width apart and flat on the floor.

B. Squeeze your heels together by pivoting on your toes and forefeet to touch your heels.

C. Hold the squeeze for a count of two. Then return your feet to the original position for a count of two.

D. Repeat this exercise for 10 repetitions 2-3 times a day.

4. Roll for Control® Exercise #4
Standing Plié (Knee Bends)

A. Stand with your feet hip width apart and your toes pointing outward.

B. Bend your knees 3-4 inches and let your knees roll out slightly for a slow count of five as you inhale.

C. Return slowly to the upright position, straightening your knees and letting your knees roll in for a slow count of five as you exhale.

D. Relax everything for a slow count of 10.

E. Repeat this exercise for 10 repetitions two times a day.

The knee-bend position with the knees rolling out brings in the obturator internus and pelvic muscles. The knee-straightening position with the knees rolling in brings in the adductor and pelvic muscles.

WEEKLY PROGRESS REPORT - WEEK THREE

Daily Activity Record Insert a slash (/) for every exercise session, P for Physiological Quieting and an F for every glass of fluid you drink.

MON	TUE	WED	THUR	FRI	SAT	SUN

Bladder/Bowel Diary

Name _____

Day_____ Date_____	Day_____ Date_____
6-8am _____	6-8am _____
8-10 _____	8-10 _____
10-12 _____	10-12 _____
12-2pm _____	12-2pm _____
2-4 _____	2-4 _____
4-6 _____	4-6 _____
6-8 _____	6-8 _____
8-10 _____	8-10 _____
10-12 _____	10-12 _____
overnight _____	overnight _____
*pads used _____	*pads used _____
comments _____	comments _____

T=toilet   F-8oz. fluid
L=small leak   *=caffeinated
A=large leak   P=pad
B=bowel movement
BC=bowel movement constipation
BD= bowel movement diarrhea

BEYOND KEGELS PROGRAM – WEEK FOUR THROUGH EIGHT

Continue the program until frequency, urgency or leaking is eliminated and toileting is every 2-4 hours during the day and bowel patterns are normalized. Then proceed to the Maintenance Plan.

1. **Lifestyle**
   A. Sleep 8-9 hours per night
   B. Drink 6-8 eight ounce glasses of noncaffeinated fluid daily.
   C. Eat fruits and vegetables to normalize bowel.
   D. Walk 30 minutes per day.
   E. Positive Self Statements- PSSTs daily

2. **Physiological Quieting**
   #1 Physiological Quieting® CD nightly.
   #2 Diaphragmatic Breathing & Handwarming hourly.

3. **Roll for Control® Exercises 2-3 times daily, 10 repetitions each.**
   #1 Relaxed Awareness 30 Seconds
   #2-O Roll Out- Obturator Assist Exercise
   #2-A Roll In- Adductor Assist Exercise
   #3 Heel Clicks
   #4 Standing Plié- Knee Bends

4. **Record data weekly.**

MAINTENANCE PLAN

1. Sleep 8-9 hours per night.

2. Adequate fluids and minimal caffeine, alcohol or other bladder irritants. Fruits and vegetables as appropriate for normal bowel pattern.

3. Walk 30 minutes per day.

4. Physiological Quieting®
Use diaphragmatic breathing and handwarming daily.
Use CD as need at night.

5. Roll for Control® Exercises – Roll out and Roll In Exercises
Perform 10 repetitions of each before you get up in the morning or in bed at night. Perform the exercises with out the ball and band some of the time.

6. Roll for Control® Exercises – Standing Plié
Perform 10 repetitions morning or night.

7. Roll for Control® Exercise- Heel Clicks
Perform 10 repetitions morning or night.

8. Wonder W'edge™ Inversion 1-2 times/day for three to five minutes.

Congratulations!
You have completed your personal program for bladder and bowel health.

Now help a friend by giving them information or a personal care kit.

COMPARISION DATA RECORD

Bladder Record	Base line	Week One	Week Two	Week Three	Week Four	Week Five	Week Six	Week Seven	Week Eight	Baseline vs. Final
# Leaks/night										
# Leaks/day										
Bowel Movements										
Toileting Freq/day										
Toileting Freq/night										
Fluids Intake										
Pads Use										

Glossary

Anal Sphincter Two rings of muscles surrounding the rectum and anus which help to control passage of bowel movements.

Anus Muscular opening at the end of the rectum is the outlet for solid waste.

Behavior Therapy Treatment involving conditioning.

Benign Prostatic Hyperplasia (BPH) Condition characterized by growth of a benign tumor inside the prostate, often resulting in voiding difficulties. Also known as benign prostate hypertrophy.

Benign Tumor Non-cancerous tissue growth that cannot spread to other areas of the body.

Biopsy Diagnostic procedure of surgically removing a tissue sample from the body and analyzing it microscopically for abnormal tissue growth.

Bladder Muscular organ located inside the pelvis for temporary storage of urine.

Blood Count Test used to determine the number and ratio of red and white blood cells and platelets in an individual's blood. Abnormal numbers can indicate infection, anemia, or cancer.

Blood Tests Samples of individual's blood that can include a blood count, sedimentation rate, glucose level, cholesterol and triglyceride levels, and special tests for prostate cancer (PSA and PAP tests).

Bulbocavernous Muscle One of three muscles of the urogenital diaphragm.

Cancer Disease characterized by uncontrolled cell growth and spread of cells to other parts of the body. Cell growth can crowd out or interfere with normal cell function causing organ dysfunction and death of healthy cells.

Castration Removal of testes or elimination of testicular function with antiandrogen drugs.

Catheter Flexible tube inserted into a body part such as the urethra (in male or female) to empty the bladder of urine.

Cervix Lower portion of the uterus that connects with the vagina.

Chemotherapy Cancer treatment using potent drugs that attack and destroy tissue cells and interfere with the cells multiplying. These drugs are either injected or taken orally.

Clitoris Organ of female orgasm.

Collagen Chemical substance injected into the internal urinary sphincter region to treat incontinence.

Colon Lower portion of large intestine leading to the rectum.

Computerized Tomography (CT scan) A computer-enhanced X-ray technique used to examine soft body tissue.

Congestion Buildup of fluid in an area of the body that often causes pain, ie., prostate congestion.

Constipation Hard, dry, and firm bowel movements that are difficult to pass and less frequent than normal.

Contraindication Side effects of a medical treatment which would indicate the treatment is more harmful than the intended benefits.

Cryosurgery Surgery that utilizes extreme cold to destroy undesired tissue.

Cystocele Bulging of the bladder into the anterior vaginal wall.

Cystogram Tube with light and a viewing lens at the end, which is inserted into the urethra to examine the urethra, bladder, and prostate gland.

Cystoscopy Diagnostic procedure for urological examination allowing viewing inside the urethra and bladder.

Diagnosis Determination through observation or scientific tests of the existence of symptoms of medical disorders.

Diuretic Any drug, food, or beverage that promotes increased urine excretion.

Encopresis Uncontrolled passage of bowel movement or smears of fecal material into underwear or inappropriate places by an individual over the age of four.

Enterocele A bulging of the pouch of Douglas into the posterior vaginal wall.

Enuresis Involuntary loss of urine, during sleep termed "nocturnal."

Episiotomy Surgical incision into the perineum between the vagina and anus to ease childbirth through the vagina.

Estrogen Hormone contributing to female sex characteristics, produced in female ovaries and male testicles, in adrenal glands, and fat.

Functional Incontinence Physical disability or mental confusion leading to inability to void in an appropriate place.

Hormone Chemical substances made in endocrine glands and essential for human biological processes.

Hormonal Therapy Treatment based on administering hormone or chemical substances that block the action of other hormones. Hormonal therapy blocks action of male hormones that promote tumor growth.

Hysterectomy Surgical removal of the uterus.

Iliococcygeal Muscle One of the muscles forming the pelvic diaphragm/levator ani muscle group.

Impotence Inability of a man to achieve or maintain an erection of sufficient duration.

Incontinence Loss of urinary control.

Intravenous Pyelogram (IVP) Diagnostic procedure to examine the urinary system with X-ray after injecting image-enhancing substances into the bloodstream.

Introitus The external vaginal opening.

Ischiocavernous Muscle One of three muscles forming the urogenital diaphragm.

Ischiococcygeal Muscle Also known as the puborectalis muscle, one of the three muscles forming the pelvic diaphragm/levator ani muscle group.

Kegel Exercises Pelvic muscle exercise to decrease or eliminate incontinence.

Kidneys Two glandular organs that separate waste products from the blood.

Magnetic Resonance Imaging (MRI) Diagnostic technique using an electromagnetic field and computer analysis, which effectively evaluates soft body tissue, such as the prostate and bladder.

Menopause Cessation of menstruation, usually occurs in the late 40's or early 50's.

Orchiectomy Surgical removal of testicles.

Overflow Incontinence Temporary inability to void, followed by uncontrollable urine flow, associated with over-distension of the bladder.

Pelvic Diaphragm The levator ani muscle group.

Pelvic Muscles General term referring to the muscles of the pelvic diaphragm and urogenital diaphragm as one unit, sometimes referred to as the pelvic floor muscles.

Penis The male organ used for urination.

Perineum/Perineal Muscles Area of muscle and tissue between the vagina or scrotum and anus.

Prostate Firm, muscular gland that surrounds the urethra in males.

Prostatectomy Surgical removal of all or part of the prostate gland.

Prostatitis Infection of the prostate; can be acute or chronic.

Pubic Bone Lower front part of the pelvis.

Pubic Symphysis Where the two pubic bones meet.

Pubococcygeal Muscle One of three muscles forming the pelvic diaphragm/levator ani muscle group.

Pudendal Nerve Innervates the external urethral and anal sphincters and the pelvic and urogenital diaphragm muscles; it is part of the voluntary nervous system.

Radiation Therapy X-ray or other high-energy radiation treatment to destroy malignant, cancerous tissue.

Radical Prostatectomy Complete removal of the prostate gland, often used to treat prostate cancer.

Rectocele A bulging of the rectum into the posterior vaginal wall.

Rectum Final several inches of the intestines below the colon and above the anus.

Reflex Incontinence Loss of urine due to hyperactivity of the bladder muscle and/or involuntary urethral relaxation in the absence of the sensation associated with the desire to urinate. This occurs in neurogenic disorders.

Sphincter Circular muscle that tightens and relaxes to control the flow of urine from the urethra. There are internal and external urethral and anal sphincters.

Stress Incontinence Loss of small amounts of urine with increased intra-abdominal pressure during coughing, sneezing, laughing, jumping, running.

Testicles Two glands that produce sperm and sex hormones including testosterone in males (testes).

Testosterone Male sex hormone that is responsible for male sexual characteristics.

Trigone Base of bladder, near bladder neck that is most sensitive area of bladder.

Tumor Body mass caused by abnormal cell growth.

Ultrasound High-frequency sound waves used for medical diagnosis and treatment. An ultrasound scan (sonogram) is sound waves reflected off internal organs to produce computer-enhanced pictures of the bladder, prostate, and urethra.

Urethra Tube connecting the bladder to the outside through which urine is released.

Urethrocele Bulging of the urethra into the vaginal wall.

Urge Incontinence Sudden leaking of relatively large

amounts of urine when the bladder muscle contracts, overcoming the contractions of the pelvic and urogenital diaphragm and sphincter muscles.

Urinalysis Tests on urine to diagnose diseases and infections.

Urinary Retention Quantities of urine backing up in the bladder which can cause bladder and kidney damage.

Urinary Tract Infection (UTI) Inflammation or infection in the bladder.

Urogenital Diaphragm Muscles that form the platform for the clitoris; the vagina and urethra pass through it.

Urologist Physician specializing in disorders of the urinary system.

Urology Specialty area of medicine dealing with the disorder of the urinary system.

Uterine Prolapse Descent of the uterus into the vaginal canal.

Uterus Muscular hollow organ that houses the fetus during pregnancy.

Vagina Elastic canal extending from the uterine cervix to the outside. Vaginal walls usually touch but can greatly expand, such as during childbirth.

X-rays Subatomic high energy particle of short wave length that penetrate body tissues to produce photographic images for diagnostic purposes.

What Organizations Can Help?

National Association for Continence (NAFC)
www.nafc.org

The Simon Foundation for Continence
www.simonfoundation.org

American Urogynecology Society
www.augs.org

Section on Women's Health
American Physical Therapy Association
www.womenshealthapta.org

US Too International, Inc
www.ustoo.com

National Institute of Diabetes and Digestive and Kidney
Diseases - National Institute of Health
www.niddk.nih.gov

About the Author

Janet A. Hulme, M.A., P.T., has been a physical therapist for over 36 years. She lectures extensively throughout the country on women's health, chronic pain, and incontinence. Janet has been certified in biofeedback, perineometry and childbirth education. She has been a professor and private practice clinician performing research and involved in developing new clinical protocols. She is the author of numerous books, DVD's and CD's in her specialty areas. She lives in Missoula, Montana when she is not traveling. You can contact her at www.phoenixcore.com.

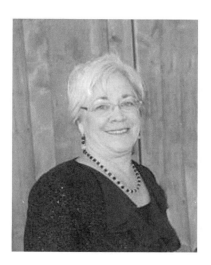

ORDER FORM

Beyond Kegels: Fabulous Four (Book 1)	____@$14.95 = $_____
Beyond Kegels: Personal Care Kit	____@$39.00 = $_____
Geriatric Incontinence	____@$24.95 = $_____
Bladder & Bowel Issues for Kids	____@$14.95 = $_____
Roll for Control Exercise DVD	____@$24.95 = $_____
Wonder W'edge	____@$31.95 = $_____
Physiological Quieting CD	____@$15.00 = $_____
Fibromyalgia: A Handbook for Self Care & Treatment	____@$14.95 = $_____
Pelvic Pain and Low Back Pain	____@$24.95 = $_____
	Subtotal = $_____
	Shipping/Handling = $_____

Total Cost of Order = $_____

Postage & Handling	
If your order is:	
up to $15.00	Add $ 3.50
$ 15.01 - $ 30.00	Add $ 5.00
$ 30.01 - $ 50.00	Add $ 7.50
$ 50.01 - $ 75.00	Add $ 9.00
$ 75.01 - $100.00	Add $ 10.50
$100.01 - $150.00	Add $12.00
$150.01 - $200.00	Add $13.50
$200.00 - $250.00	Add $16.50
$250.01 - $300.00	Add $19.50

Send Check/Credit card Money Order in U.S. Funds To:

Phoenix Publishing
P.O. Box 8231
Missoula, MT 59807

or call us at 1-800-549-8371

or order online at:
www.phoenixpub.com

We appreciate and thank you for your order!

Name_____

Address_____

City_____State_____Zip_____

Telephone (____) _____ Fax (____) _____

Acct. #_____Exp. Date____ /____

☐ MasterCard ☐ VISA Signature_____